Nutrition Logic:

Food First, Supplements Second

MARIE DUNFORD,
PHD, RD

Published by Pink Robin Publishing

Dunford, Marie, PhD, RD

Nutrition Logic: Food First, Supplements Second

©2003 by Marie Dunford, PhD, RD

First printing 2003

ISBN: 0-9729888-0-7

Developmental Editor: Susan Brown Zahn, PhD

Copyeditor: Jan Feeney

Graphic Designer: Nancy Loch Graphic Design & Consultation

Proofreader: Kim Thoren

Published by Pink Robin Publishing

To my husband, Greg
The light of my life and my biggest fan

CONTENTS

INTRODUCTION

Do you ever say, "I don't want to diet; I just want to eat right"? Are you so overwhelmed with information about what you should and shouldn't eat that you don't know where to begin? Do you ever wonder whether you should take a dietary supplement? If so, then this book, *Nutrition Logic: Food First, Supplements Second,* can help.

Thousands of weight-loss books are on the market, but there aren't many diet books. This is a diet (that is, a pattern of eating) book, not a weight-loss book. You will read about a positive approach to diet and learn how to eat well so that you can be healthy and stay healthy as you get older. You will focus on what you *should* eat rather than on what you *shouldn't* eat. This book also helps you decide whether you need supplements, and if you do, how much is safe to take. The information is based on scientific studies that show which foods and supplements can help prevent disease.

Because this is a diet book and not a weight-loss diet book, caloric intake is not emphasized. You will focus on the amount of calories (energy) you need for maintaining your current body weight, and you will determine whether your current weight is a healthy weight. A healthy weight is one that decreases your risk of premature death and disease, not one that is based on your appearance. You will find out why a woman who is 5'5" tall and 140 pounds is at a healthier weight than a woman of the same height who weighs 108 pounds.

This is a book for people of all weights because it focuses on balancing food intake with physical activity. If you are currently at a healthy weight, your food intake is in balance with the amount of energy required for your physical activity. Therefore, you will focus on weight stability. If you are gaining weight, the book's focus on balance helps you stop the weight gain. No matter what you weigh, it is important to focus on taking in enough food and nutrients so that you can do physical activity and improve your fitness. It's also important to recognize that heavier people who are fit are healthier than thin people who are physically unfit. The book is perfect for you if you have tried numerous weight-loss diets that have not resulted in long-term weight loss or your main goal is to eat well, not lose weight.

This is also a book for people of all cultures. The United States is a multiethnic society, and there really is no "typical" American diet. Caucasians eat sushi and Asians eat tacos. Salsa and ketchup are next to each other on the grocery store shelf. People around the world need the same essential nutrients, and for millions of years people have obtained these nutrients from local foods. Today foods are transported long distances, and you have many choices. This book helps you discover the many possible sources of nutrients, not just the well-known ones. For example, you can get vitamin C from bok choy (Chinese cabbage) as well as from oranges.

This is a nutrition book for adults without any serious disease requiring medical nutritional therapy (such as heart disease, diabetes, or kidney disease). It is based on science but written for consumers. The focus is on the consumption of types and amounts of food known to be beneficial rather than the avoidance of certain foods. By reading this book, you will learn how to get the nutrients you need from food and how to determine whether you need supplements.

Food is the vehicle by which you get the majority of your nutrients. That food generally comes from the grocery store or a restaurant, although you may have the good fortune to get some from your garden or from a roadside stand. If you choose wisely, you should be able to obtain all the nutrients you need from food. If you choose your food unwisely, you may not obtain all the required nutrients. In that case, supplementation is a reasonable alternative but usually not equal to nutrient-containing foods.

Just as food should be chosen wisely, supplements also must be chosen carefully. You might need supplements to prevent nutrient deficiencies and provide nutrients you do not obtain in your diet. But taking unneeded supplements is a waste of money and, in certain cases, can harm you. Government regulation of dietary supplements is weak, so know what you are taking and why you are taking it. To that end, this book will provide you with facts to make an informed decision.

What can you expect from this book?

- A philosophy that emphasizes food, physical activity, and possibly supplements because your good health is always the ultimate goal

- A lesson in the language of nutrition so that you can understand your body's nutrient needs and interpret food labels
- A demonstration of a pattern of eating, not a pattern of restriction

As the title reveals, the emphasis of this book is on food, which is the topic of part I. Supplements are discussed in part II. Are they safe and effective? These are vital questions. Are you ready to get started making the best decisions you can about your diet?

The *Nutrition Logic* Philosophy

Food is the primary source of nutrients. Supplements may be necessary for preventing or reversing a nutrient deficiency, and some supplements may be beneficial under other circumstances. The scientific literature is the basis for diet and supplement information, and proof of safety and effectiveness are essential. You, as a consumer, must be responsible for gathering the necessary information to make an informed decision. You must be an open-minded skeptic and make decisions while considering both the risks and the benefits.

By definition, *dietary supplement* means "to add to the diet." This assumes that careful thought has been given first to the basic diet. Adopting a nutritious diet and exercising regularly are the foundation of good health; they should be among life's daily priorities. No supplement can come close to providing the benefits that diet and exercise bring. "I don't have time to eat right" or "I don't have time to exercise" are lame excuses. We all find time to do things that are important to us. Good health is one of the most important aspects in life. If you don't believe that, just ask someone who is sick.

The idea behind this book is to know about the nutrients you need and the foods that contain those nutrients, which is a logical approach to good nutrition. Because nutrition is a complicated subject, the book includes some special features that make it easier to understand. Let's take a look.

The *Nutrition Logic* Format

Once you have the basic information about the nutrients that you need and the foods that contain those nutrients, you can build a diet that provides a sufficient amount of carbohydrates, proteins, fats, vitamins, minerals, and water. Nutrients are found naturally in food, can be added to food (through enrichment or fortification), and can be taken in the form of a dietary supplement. The advantages and disadvantages of each type of nutrient will be explained.

The following features will help you to identify nutrients that you need and the foods that contain those nutrients:

- **Take-Home Messages.** People are often confused about nutrition. The terminology can be difficult to understand, and advertising adds to the confusion. Throughout part I of this book you will find Take-Home Messages, which are short pieces of advice to think about when eating, shopping for food, and planning your diet.

- **Fabulous Foods.** Some foods contain so much of a particular nutrient that they deserve special mention. These Fabulous Foods are among the richest, naturally occurring sources known. Remember, though, that variety is a very important diet-planning concept; you should not consume one food, even a fabulous food, to the exclusion of other foods.

- **How Am I Doing So Far?** This is a major feature of the book. It's where nutrition facts are translated into food choices. The sample diets will show you how the nutrients in individual foods become part of a healthy overall diet.

- **The Big Easy.** Dietary changes are difficult to make, so tips are included that take little effort. These tips are found in appendix A.

- **Time and Money.** Surveys show that time and money are big considerations when it comes to choosing foods. Some people have more time than money; others have more money than time. Tips are given in appendix B for both circumstances.

- **Beyond the Borders.** People around the world need the same essential nutrients. For millions of years people have obtained nutrients from locally available food. You may obtain calcium by drinking cow's milk; but another person thousands of miles away may get calcium by eating small fish with bones, such as sardines. The calcium is the same regardless of whether it comes from milk or fish bones. The Beyond the Borders in appendix C introduces many different foods and gives you a chance to try a nutritious food that you might not have considered otherwise.

Use of the Word *Diet*

Your goal is to build a healthy diet. In this book, the word *diet* refers to the foods and beverages that you consume; it does not carry a negative connotation. Unfortunately in the United States, the word *diet* is usually associated with food and calorie restriction in an effort to lose weight. Thus, people talk (constantly) about "being on a diet." This usage implies that you can go "off" a diet. A diet is a pattern of eating; therefore, a person cannot go "on" or "off" a diet.

People do change their diet (pattern of eating) in an effort to lose weight. The term *weight-loss diet* should be used when calories are restricted and loss of body weight is a goal. The word *diet* still refers to a pattern of eating. But again, this book emphasizes diet, *not* weight loss.

Measuring Success

You will learn how to develop a diet that gives you all of the necessary nutrients and an adequate amount of calories to fuel activity. With this book you will not focus on weight loss as a measure of success. But how will you measure success? One measure of success is the consumption of 100% of the recommended intake of nutrients. A second measure of success is that food provides most of your nutrients. A third measure of success is that, if necessary, you can choose dietary supplements wisely based on scientific material that supports their safety and effectiveness.

Should I Not . . .?

When people ask questions about their diets, they often begin with "Should I not . . .?" Should I not eat meat? Should I not drink milk? Should I not eat sugar? But "Should I not . . .?" is the wrong question. The important question is, "If I don't . . . (eat meat, drink milk, and so on), what nutrients will I be missing and what foods will I need to eat to provide those nutrients?"

If you have been eating red meat, and you eliminate it from your diet, you will eliminate a source of protein, iron, and zinc. What foods will you include in your diet that will provide those nutrients? If you don't drink milk, how will you obtain calcium in your diet? Those are critical questions, and you need more information to be able to answer those questions. (See chapter 12 for the answers to the questions.)

Perspective

When people think about changing their diets they generally start with their present intake and try to modify it. That's not a bad idea. But it often means that people look at foods they need to eliminate from their current diets in order to be healthier. The focus can easily become one of restriction. Here's an idea from a different perspective: Begin by looking at what your body needs, and find foods to include in your diet that provide the needed nutrients. The goal is still changing your diet so that you can be healthier, but it is from the perspective of inclusion.

The concept of "building" a diet is used throughout this book. It is a diet plan based on the principles of inclusion. Include a variety of fruits and vegetables. Include a variety of whole grains. Include beans, legumes, and nuts. You will be pleasantly surprised to know that there are hundreds of tasty, healthy foods that you should include in your diet. Ready to take a look at what to include? We'll get started by looking at nutrients occurring naturally in foods or added to foods.

Chapter 1

Is There a "Perfect" Diet?

Consumers and health professionals alike are frustrated by the conflicting information they read about diet. One month everyone is talking about high-carbohydrate, low-fat diets; the next month the talk is about low-carbohydrate, high-protein diets. Much of the debate is centered on the newest weight-loss plan that has been published. But the more things change, the more they stay the same.

The concepts of a healthy diet have been remarkably consistent over the years, even if the message to consumers has not been. For years health professionals have known that fruits, vegetables, whole grains, beans, legumes, fish, nuts, and oils are healthy foods, providing high-fiber carbohydrates, proteins, heart-healthy fats, and many vitamins and minerals. Unfortunately, over the past 50 years the American diet has been moving in another direction in which low-fiber, sweetened carbohydrates; saturated fat; and salted foods predominate.

No "perfect" diet exists. There are some good guidelines to follow, but no one pattern is perfect. And there probably never will be a perfect diet. One of the reasons is the role that genetics plays. For example, in the United States about 7% of the people do not absorb dietary cholesterol very well. These people could eat four eggs every day and their blood cholesterol levels would not increase. On the other hand, some people have a genetic predisposition to readily absorb dietary cholesterol. When they eat too many high-cholesterol foods, their blood cholesterol rises to a dangerous level. So, would eggs be included as part of a perfect diet? The answer would depend on the individual.

Maybe if there were a perfect diet it would be easier, because people wouldn't have to make choices. Healthful eating means choosing a variety of foods that provide the needed nutrients. And sometimes choosing is the hard part. This book can help you make healthy choices.

Let's take a look at where we can get the nutrients we need.

Take-Home Message: Think of your diet as a pattern of eating, not as a pattern of restriction.

Where Do We Get Nutrients?

Nutrients come from three sources: They exist naturally in food, they are added to food during processing, and they exist in supplements.

An orange is a food, and a calcium pill is a supplement; but what about a processed food like calcium-fortified orange juice? The market is exploding with processed foods that have added nutrients, and you must be able to make decisions about consuming them. An orange contains vitamin C, and milk is a source of calcium; so people who consume enough of these foods can obtain these two nutrients through food alone—the recommended approach of food first, supplements second. Calcium-fortified orange juice is a food–supplement blend. The addition of calcium does not in any way detract from the benefit of the orange juice. In fact, the acids in the orange juice enhance the absorption of the calcium. This processed food would be recommended for someone who cannot tolerate milk and lacks dietary calcium. But what about someone who drinks a glass of orange juice and takes a calcium supplement? There really isn't much difference in the nutrient levels, although the calcium-fortified orange juice may be more convenient. In this case, the orange juice and calcium supplement would be equivalent to the calcium-fortified orange juice.

Unfortunately, judging most of the processed foods on the market is not as simple as the calcium-fortified orange juice example. There are enriched and fortified foods. There are functional foods, designer foods, and nutraceuticals. Choosing a nutritious diet has certainly become more complicated, and the consumer is left to figure it all out. Let's take a look at what's behind those claims of "fortified" and "enriched" that are emblazoned across cereal boxes and bread wrappers.

Adding Nutrients to Foods: Fortified, Enriched, Functional, and Designer Foods

Food has always been a way for people to obtain nutrients. Before the discovery and isolation of nutrients in the laboratory, food stood on the merit of the nutrients it contained naturally. People use the word *naturally* to mean that the nutrients were put there by nature, such as the vitamin C in an orange when it is picked from the tree. The nutrient content of foods began to change when food processing became widespread. When raw foods are processed, nutrients may be lost. Thus, when whole-grain wheat is processed into white flour, nutrients that were originally in the whole grain are removed. But processing may also add nutrients to foods.

There is a strong argument for getting the nutrients that occur naturally in food. After all, people wouldn't have been able to survive for millions of years if foods couldn't provide the nutrients they needed to live. Scientists have found that nutrients that occur naturally in foods are in perfect proportion to each other, such as the ratio of calcium to phosphorous in milk or the ratio of potassium to sodium in fruits and vegetables. Foods don't naturally contain toxic levels of vitamins or minerals, and the natural sugars in fruits are diluted with water and accompanied by vitamins, minerals, and other biologically active compounds. In some ways it is intuitive that Mother Nature knows best.

Although it is true that people have survived for millions of years with only the nutrients that occur naturally in food, it is also true that people suffered from malnutrition. In the United States, nutrient deficiencies were so widespread by the 1940s that a law was passed that allowed nutrients to be added to food. The reason for the law was related to the changing dietary habits of Americans at that time. White bread had become so widely accepted that it was a staple in the diet of many people. The processing of whole grains into white bread reduced the amount of thiamin, riboflavin, niacin, and iron in the white flour; deficiencies of these vitamins and minerals were common. Enrichment (restoring nutrients lost during processing) and fortification (adding nutrients in amounts not previously found in a food), really forms of supplementation, had begun in this country.

A close look at the foods consumed in the United States helps us realize that all of us consume foods that contain supplements. We receive several nutrients via the enrichment and fortification processes. A 1996 amendment to the law from the 1940s requires that folate be added to flour as well as thiamin, riboflavin, niacin, and iron. Folate fortification is a good example of how health is enhanced when nutrients are added to food.

Folate is a vitamin necessary for preventing neural tube defects in newborns. During the first few weeks of pregnancy, the cells of the fetus divide rapidly; if sufficient folate is not available, then the tissue around the spinal cord may not fully develop. Folate is found in fruits and green leafy vegetables, but most women of childbearing age do not consume enough folate. Many women change their eating habits once they know that they are pregnant, but the need for folate is great before and just after conception, a time when most women do not know that they are pregnant. The addition of folate to flour is expected to reduce the incidence of neural tube defects by 50%.

Adding vitamin D is another example of the benefits of fortification. A lack of vitamin D causes rickets, a bone disease that results in bowed legs and other abnormal bone development. Milk in the United States is fortified with vitamin D, so the prevalence of rickets is rare here. The amount of vitamin D added is carefully calculated because vitamin D is the most toxic of the vitamins.

Other products are fortified with nutrients that would otherwise be lacking in some diets. Many vegetarian products, notably soy milk, are fortified with vitamin B_{12} which is found naturally only in animal products. Orange juice and soy milk are fortified with calcium. A good argument can be made that enrichment and fortification of food have helped prevent nutrient deficiencies.

Since the 1940s a pattern has emerged: Nutrient deficiencies that lead to diseases are offset by the addition of the missing nutrient to foods that are widely consumed. This practice has been effective in eliminating many nutrient deficiencies in the United States. A close look at ready-to-eat cereal reveals that many such cereals contain 10 or more added nutrients and some advertise 100% Daily Value of 12 vitamins and minerals. (*Daily Value* is a term used on food labels and is an estimate of the amount of certain nutrients you need each day. It is not as specific for your age and gender as the Dietary Reference Intakes, on which the Daily Value is based. Dietary Reference Intakes are found in appendix O.) The choice of some cereals is really a choice of food plus a multivitamin and mineral supplement.

The new century has brought more products that include 100% Daily Value for various nutrients. Energy bars, a popular product on the market today, seem to mirror the cereal market. Energy bars contain added vitamins and minerals, and manufacturers use the addition of these nutrients as a prominent part of their advertising. There is even a product called vitamin water. Some scientists are concerned that people could easily exceed recommended upper intake levels because of the number of foods that are fortified with many nutrients.

You may wonder whether processed foods are good or bad. They are both. Some processed foods are beneficial because they provide nutrients that would be difficult to obtain otherwise (such as iron and folate), and our nutritional status and health are better because of food processing. We have nutritious foods available all year. Foods that could spoil are preserved safely. We don't want to go back to the days of nutrient deficiencies.

On the other hand, processed foods may have added ingredients that people already overconsume, such as sugar and fat. Manufacturers may add more sugar, salt, or fat than you would add if you prepared the food. The processing also may change the natural balance of the nutrients. The more a food is processed, the more likely it is that nutrients have been lost. Processed foods are available year-round and may encourage people to eat less fresh food.

So processed foods are both harmful and beneficial to your goal of obtaining the nutrients that you need to be healthy. As a general rule, the less a food is processed, the more naturally occurring nutrients it contains.

The market continues to expand: Functional foods, designer foods, and nutraceuticals are among the new choices as people look for ways to combat chronic diseases. Chronic diseases are degenerative diseases that get progressively worse. Heart disease, cancer, osteoporosis, and diabetes are examples of chronic diseases. Once you get a chronic disease you will live with it for the rest of your life. Good nutrition has been shown to prevent or delay the onset of chronic disease. Eating properly also helps to slow the progression of these diseases, which makes nutrition vitally important because people are living longer. Functional and designer foods are conventional foods that have nutrients added to protect against chronic diseases. Nutraceuticals are nutrients in foods (or supplements) that may have a medicinal effect. Examples of these foods are listed in appendix E. No standard definitions exist for any of these terms, and the Food and Drug

Administration (FDA) does little to regulate these foods. Simply stated, these are foods that are modified with ingredients known to confer health benefits.

Whatever they are called, these foods are not created to combat malnutrition from the lack of nutrients; rather, they are created to provide nutrients to prevent or delay the onset of chronic diseases. In some cases a nutrient that is naturally in the food is added so that the food will have a greater concentration of that nutrient. An example is the addition of calcium to milk, resulting in a product known as "high-calcium" milk. In other cases, nutrients never occurring naturally in a product are added, which is the case in calcium-fortified orange juice. In both cases the calcium is added to prevent or delay the onset of osteoporosis.

An emerging category is herbal foods. Herbs, one type of dietary supplement, are added to foods because of their medicinal (healing) properties. The FDA considers herbs neither foods nor drugs so they are not regulated as foods and drugs are. Beverages, soups, and bars that contain herbs such as echinacea, ginseng, ginkgo, kava, and saw palmetto are available. You must be aware of the amount of herbs and the risks and benefits of the herbs in these foods because there is no government approval process before these foods appear on the market. Herbal foods are covered in greater depth in part II of this book.

Now that we've taken a look at the sources of nutrients, how can we translate this information into diet planning?

Nutrients That the Body Needs

An obvious starting point in planning a diet is to know the nutrients that your body needs. Although there is much yet to be discovered about human nutrition and its relationship to health, we do know some of the essentials. Generally, the human body requires six classes of nutrients: carbohydrates, proteins, fats, vitamins, minerals, and water. Each category contains even more specific nutrients that the human body requires. In the protein category, for example, there are 20 required amino acids. Nine of these amino acids must be obtained from food because your body cannot manufacture them. At least 14 vitamins and 21 minerals are essential. Knowing all the nutrients that your body needs becomes complicated very quickly.

To simplify matters, nutritionists have devised various methods to help people plan their diets. The most common methods involve grouping foods together that contain approximately the same amount of nutrients. The best-known tools are the Food Guide Pyramid and the Food Exchange Lists. It is difficult to reduce a complicated matter to a simple concept, so it is no surprise that the Food Guide Pyramid and other such methods are oversimplified. Vegetables are grouped together into one category, even though there is a big difference between broccoli and iceberg lettuce in terms of their respective amounts of nutrients.

People have become more sophisticated about nutrition, and they need more sophisticated information. The more sophisticated information is contained in the Dietary Reference Intakes (DRI) in appendix O. The DRI, which expands on and replaces the Recommended Dietary Allowances (RDA), can help you plan and assess your diet. Dietary Reference Intakes have been established for 14 vitamins and 12 minerals but are not available for all nutrients. The DRI are an estimate of the amount of a nutrient you need to take in to prevent a deficiency and to reduce the risk for chronic diseases such as heart disease, some kinds of cancer, or osteoporosis. Dietary Reference Intakes are not perfect, but they are a good guideline.

As important as vitamins and minerals are, they aren't the only focus of the diet. Carbohydrates, proteins, and fats are very important because they provide energy to fuel the body. Having enough energy to carry out your daily activities is one of your body's top priorities. Many of the vitamins and minerals help process the energy provided by the carbohydrates, proteins, and fats. The amount of nutrients you consume depends in part on the amount of food you eat.

Portion Size

Food portion refers to the size of a serving. In some cases the person consuming the food determines the portion size, such as when spooning out a helping from a casserole dish. In other cases other people may influence the portion size. For example, a parent may say that the portion a child selects is too much (chocolate cake) or too little (vegetables). Much of the time the portion size is predetermined, such as the amount of food served at a restaurant or the size of a vending machine item.

Since the 1970s portion sizes of food have increased dramatically in the United States. The typical bagel was 2 to 3 ounces then, but now bagels are closer to 7 ounces. A fast-food hamburger was thin and small (about 3 ounces) compared to burgers today: Single patties can be 6 to 8 ounces, or multiple small patties are featured. The size of soft drinks is one of the most dramatic examples. The 10-ounce soft drink bottle so familiar in the 1970s has been replaced with larger cups, some holding 64 ounces.

No one is forcing you to eat more than you want, but whether you do eat the entire portion served can be a dilemma. Some people hate to waste food, and they feel guilty if they don't finish what has been served. Others hate to waste money, so they don't want to throw away food that they have paid for. Some are creatures of habit, and they are used to eating the amount set in front of them. They typically don't make conscious choices about portion size. One guideline for food intake is "eat when you're hungry and stop when you're full." If you apply this guideline, your degree of fullness determines how much you eat, not the size of the portion.

"Eat when you're hungry and stop when you're full" may sound like easy advice to follow, but many people aren't aware of when they are full because they haven't paid much attention to fullness cues. Slow down your eating by taking small bites, chewing each bite several times, and sipping water between each bite. Pay attention to your level of fullness at various points in a meal. You may *find* that you are full even though there is still food on the plate. Feelings of hunger and fullness are less extreme when you don't let yourself get too hungry. Ravenous hunger often means overconsuming food because the body's fullness feedback system takes some time to work (about 20 minutes). One way to avoid ravenous hunger is to eat when you begin to feel hungry.

In this country the concern over increasing portion size is focused on the amount of excess nutrients that people consume as a result of eating large portions. Naturally, large portions of food contain more calories than smaller portions; many of those foods contain a lot of sugar and fat, nutrients whose intake should be moderate. The amount of food that you eat should be in balance with the amount of activity and exercise you perform. When the standard portion is large, it is likely that it contains too many calories, too much fat, and too much sugar for the average adult who, in the United States, is likely to be physically inactive. Oversized adult portions eaten routinely by children are thought to be one factor of childhood obesity.

Since the 1970s portion sizes have also become more quantified. This has been a result of nutrition labeling laws. In order for a label to indicate the amount of nutrients a food contains, a portion size must appear. The portion size is referred to as serving size on the label. Serving sizes are given in household measurements like cups, ounces, and teaspoons. Looking at the serving size used on a food label will help you to get an idea of a reasonably sized portion. We'll spend some time looking at food labeling later.

Right now, let's take the first step in building a diet. We begin by looking at what your body needs and find foods to include in your diet that provide the needed nutrients. A good starting point is establishing the goal of obtaining a healthy amount of carbohydrates.

Chapter 2

Complex Carbohydrate Foods

Carbohydrates comprise sugars and starches. The emphasis should be on starchy foods because they contain complex carbohydrates and fiber. Most Americans do not consume enough starches but overconsume sugars.

A frequent question is, "How many complex carbohydrates and fiber do I need?" The simple answer to this question is **300 grams of mostly complex carbohydrates and 25 grams of fiber daily.** It is also recommended that adults consume **three servings of whole grains per day.**

The recommended 300 grams of carbohydrates is based on the Daily Value for a 2,000-calorie diet because there is no Dietary Reference Intake established. Many men consume 300 grams of carbohydrate per day, but many women do not. Some people prefer to consume fewer carbohydrates and more proteins, and such diets can also be adequate. The minimum recommended amount of carbohydrates per day for men and nonpregnant women is 130 grams. The minimum recommendation is based on the amount of glucose (the end point in the body of all carbohydrates) needed by the brain.

Complex carbohydrates are found in starchy foods made from grains (grasses that bear seeds). Wheat, corn, and rice are among the best known. Rye, oats, barley, and millet are also grains. Wheat is made into flour, and the flour is made into other products, notably breads and cereals. Other grains are also made into flour (e.g., cornmeal) or eaten cooked (such as rice and oatmeal).

The most healthful grains are whole grains, which contain the endosperm, the germ, and the bran. When whole grains are processed, the germ and the bran are removed, leaving only the endosperm, which is ground to make flour. The removal of the germ and the bran through processing causes many nutrients, including fiber, several

B vitamins, trace minerals, and many phytochemicals, to be lost. Consumption of whole grains reduces the risk for heart disease and stomach, colon, breast, and prostate cancer. Unfortunately, only 13% of adult Americans eat one or more servings of whole grains daily.

Bread is an important source of carbohydrates in the diets of many people. But all breads are not created equal. Flour that is minimally processed contains the most nutrients, including the most fiber. Thus, whole-grain breads, which are dark and heavy, are a rich source of nutrients. However, most of the breads on the grocery store shelves are not whole grain because consumers in the United States have expressed a preference for more refined flours and white bread.

Take-Home Message: Eat more whole-grain breads and cereals— in other words, breads and cereals that have been processed the least.

As stated earlier, when people in the United States began to eat white bread instead of whole-grain bread, their diets suffered. The refining of the whole-grain flour to white flour resulted in the substantial loss (nearly 75%) of iron, thiamin, and riboflavin and nearly all (98%) of the niacin. In 1942 a law was passed that required iron, thiamin, riboflavin, and niacin to be added to refined flour (a process known as enrichment). The act was amended in 1996 to include folate, which is also lost in the processing.

Because of the enrichment process, white bread has slightly more iron, thiamin, riboflavin, niacin, and folate than whole-grain bread. Unfortunately, some nutrients that are lost are not restored. Laws do not require vitamin B_6, fiber, magnesium, and zinc to be included in the enrichment process; these nutrients are present in much greater amounts in whole-grain bread than in white bread. Only 5% of grain products in the United States are whole-grain products, so it is not surprising that surveys show that many U.S. adults fail to meet recommended intakes of vitamin B_6, fiber, magnesium, and zinc. So the best bread choice is whole-grain bread.

THE CASE FOR EATING WHOLE-GRAIN BREAD

Nutrient	50 grams (about 2 slices) whole-grain bread	50 grams (almost 2 slices) enriched white bread
Carbohydrate (grams)	18	24
Iron (milligrams)	1.33	1.45
Thiamin (milligrams)	.16	.20
Riboflavin (milligrams)	.13	.19
Niacin (milligrams)	1.68	1.75
Folate (micrograms)	31	44
Vitamin B$_6$ (milligrams)	.13	.02
Fiber (grams)	3	1
Magnesium (milligrams)	21	9
Zinc (milligrams)	.49	.29

The gray area in the chart indicates which type of bread has more of a particular nutrient. Enriched white bread has slightly more iron, thiamin, riboflavin, niacin, and folate because of the amount that is added according to the law. When compared to enriched white bread, whole-grain bread has 96% of the niacin, 92% of the iron, 80% of the thiamin, 70% of the folate, and 68% of the riboflavin. These are still respectable amounts. In other words, both whole-grain and white breads are considered good sources of these nutrients, but white bread has more of these nutrients.

The situation changes dramatically for those nutrients not covered by enrichment laws. When compared to whole-grain bread, white bread has only 15% of the vitamin B$_6$, 33% of the fiber, 43% of the magnesium, and 59% of the zinc. These amounts are not as respectable. For these nutrients, whole-grain bread is considered a good source, but white bread is not.

Whole Grains

Now you know that bread is a good source of complex carbohydrates and that whole-grain bread contains more nutrients than white bread. But you may not eat much bread in your diet. Bagels, tortillas, high-fiber cereals, rice, and pasta noodles are also good sources of complex carbohydrates and fiber (see the following chart). The Beyond the Borders section in appendix C lists more complex carbohydrate foods. Choose a variety of carbohydrate sources and try to include three servings of whole grains every day.

SOURCES OF COMPLEX CARBOHYDRATES AND FIBER

Food	Carbohydrate (grams)	Fiber (grams)	Whole grain
1 slice whole-grain bread	18	2	✔
1 slice wheat bread	13	2	
1 slice white bread	15	1	
Whole-wheat bagel 3½ inches in diameter	38	3	✔
Bagel 3½ inches in diameter	38	2	
Whole-wheat English muffin (both halves)	27	4	✔
English muffin (both halves)	26	2	
Whole-wheat tortilla (8 inches)	27	3	✔
Flour tortilla (8 inches)	27	2	
1 cup Maypo (cooked cereal)	29	5	✔
1 cup cooked oatmeal or two ½-cup packages	25	4	✔
1 cup 40% Bran Flakes	32	7	✔
1 cup Grape Nuts Flakes	32	4	✔
1 cup Shredded Wheat	35	4	✔
½ cup cooked brown rice	23	2	✔
½ cup cooked wild rice	17	1.5	✔
½ cup cooked white rice	22	.5	
1 cup cooked whole-wheat spaghetti noodles	37	6	✔
1 cup cooked spaghetti noodles	40	4	
1 low-fat granola bar	19	1	

One confusing aspect of choosing whole-grain foods is the terms on the labels. Wheat flour is different from whole-wheat flour. The term *wheat flour* on the label means that the flour is made from the grain wheat as opposed to corn or other grains. Bread that contains white flour made from wheat can be labeled *wheat bread* but it cannot be labeled *whole-wheat bread*. *Unbleached* and brown refer to color, not to whole-grain status; and *stone-ground* refers to the milling process. Look for the terms *whole-grain* or *whole-wheat*. Remember that only 5% of all grain products in the United States are whole grains, so sometimes it is not easy to find them on the grocery store shelves.

In 1999 the FDA allowed products that contain more than 50% whole grains (by weight) and had fewer than 3 grams of fat per serving to carry a "Whole Grains Health Claim." These foods can state on the label, "Diets rich in whole-grain foods and other plant foods and low in total fat, saturated fat, and cholesterol may help reduce the risk of heart disease and certain cancers." If this statement is on the label, the food is a whole-grain food; but whole-grain foods are not required to have this label. Also, some whole-grain products have more than 3 grams of fat per serving and don't qualify for the health claim because of their fat content.

Beans and Legumes

As you can see from the following chart, beans and legumes are excellent sources of complex carbohydrates and fiber. It's puzzling why people in the United States don't eat more beans and legumes. From a nutritional perspective they are packed with nutrients: complex carbohydrates, fiber, proteins, several vitamins, iron, and other minerals. On top of that, they are cheap. So why don't more people eat beans and legumes? One reason might be that people don't know what beans and legumes are, and they are often afraid to try foods that are unfamiliar. Another reason might be that people don't know how to prepare them, or they think that preparation time is too long. Whatever your reasons for not eating beans and legumes, try to include them in your diet.

BEANS AND LEGUMES

Food	Carbohydrate (grams)	Fiber (grams)
½ cup cooked black beans	20	7
½ cup canned pork and beans	25	6
½ cup cooked split peas	21	8
½ cup cooked lentils	20	8

Legumes are usually from the plant genus *Phaseolus*. They are plants that have a double-seamed pod that contains a single row of beans (seeds). Legumes are interesting plants because they get their nutrients both from the soil and from the air. Bacteria in the roots of legumes take nitrogen from the air and add it to the plant's seeds. Nitrogen is needed by the plant to form proteins.

Examples of legumes include black-eyed peas, garbanzo beans (also known as chickpeas), kidney beans, lentils, lima beans, northern beans, red beans, soybeans, and split peas. You can find them in the grocery store in several places. One place is usually next to the rice, where they are sold in packages as dried beans. These beans are cheap and last for a long time, but they need to be soaked, cooked, and seasoned before they're eaten. The exception to the long preparation time are lentils and split peas, which require no soaking and take about 30 minutes to cook.

Take-Home Message: Eat more beans and legumes. They're cheap, convenient, and nutritious.

Legumes also can be found in the canned vegetable section. Some of the cans contain just the beans (such as a can of garbanzo beans that you can open and put on a salad), whereas other cans have seasonings added such as with baked beans (white beans that have been cooked in tomato sauce). A few, such as lima beans, can also be found in the frozen foods section.

The dried beans and peas described previously are different from green beans and green peas that are commonly consumed as vegetables in the United States. Green beans and green peas belong to a category called *edible-pod beans* and do not have the same nutrient content as dried beans and peas, which are from plants known as *fresh-shelled beans*. Just remember that from the nutrition perspective green beans and green peas fall into the vegetable category.

How Am I Doing So Far?

At this point it is time to translate knowledge into practice. You know that you need about 300 grams of mostly complex carbohydrates and 25 grams of fiber per day. It is also recommended that you consume three servings of whole grains daily. Let's build a diet that includes some of the foods already mentioned and see how close it comes to meeting the requirements. Remember that this is only the first step, and this diet is only a skeleton.

Meet Anna, who is 26 years old and works as an accountant in an office. She lives alone in an apartment and considers herself an average cook. Anna chooses whole-grain toast in the morning, split pea soup and a bagel at lunch, a granola bar for a snack, and a bean burrito with tortilla chips for dinner. Let's see how much carbohydrate, fiber, and whole grains these foods provide.

ANNA'S FOOD CHOICES:
CARBOHYDRATE, FIBER AND WHOLE GRAIN FOODS

Food	Carbohydrate (grams)	Fiber (grams)	Whole grain
2 slices whole-grain toast	24	4	2 servings
1 cup split pea soup (add water to dehydrated soup)	21	3	
3½-inch bagel	38	2	
Granola bar	19	1	
2 flour tortillas	54	4	
½ cup pinto beans	22	7	
15 tortilla chips	17	1	1 serving
TOTAL SO FAR	195	22	3 servings

The diet so far provides approximately 195 grams of carbohydrates, 22 grams of fiber, and 3 servings of whole grains. These are very respectable amounts.

Of course, not everyone likes the same foods, so let's build another diet using different foods. Ellen is 45 years old and married with two teenaged children. She works as a sales associate in a large department store. Ellen doesn't have much time in the morning, so she eats two packages of instant oatmeal using water that she has heated in the microwave. She orders a baked potato at the potato bar in the shopping mall where she works and eats pretzels as a snack. Spaghetti and French bread are part of a quick and easy dinner for the entire family, and popcorn is a favorite after-dinner snack.

ELLEN'S FOOD CHOICES:
CARBOHYDRATE, FIBER AND WHOLE GRAIN FOODS

Food	Carbohydrate (grams)	Fiber (grams)	Whole Grain
1 cup instant oatmeal	36	4	2 servings
Baked potato with skin (approximately 7 oz)	51	5	
10 Dutch Twist pretzels	47	2	
1 cup spaghetti noodles	40	4	
2 slices French bread	26	2	
1 cup microwave popcorn	4	1	1 serving
TOTAL SO FAR	204	18	3 servings

This diet so far provides 204 grams of carbohydrates, 18 grams of fiber, and 3 servings of whole grains. Although the amount of fiber is not quite as much as in the first example, this diet is still a good start toward meeting the recommended goals.

It is interesting to note that so far these diets consist of only six or seven foods. Complex carbohydrates form the foundation of these diets. Let's build on these foundations by adding protein foods.

Chapter 3

Protein Foods

The word *protein* comes from the Greek word *proteios,* which means "of prime importance." Because protein foods are so easy to come by in the United States, we sometimes forget how important this nutrient is in our diet. Looking at pictures of starving children and adults can quickly remind us what happens when people do not eat adequate protein and calories.

Proteins are made up of amino acids. Of the 20 amino acids that adults need, 9 of them must be provided by the diet because your body cannot make them. They are termed *essential amino acids.* The remaining 11 amino acids are manufactured by your body.

Proteins from animal sources contain all the essential amino acids in the proper quantities and proportions. Meat (beef, lamb, and pork), poultry (chicken, duck, goose, guinea, pigeon, and turkey), fish, milk, cheese, and eggs are examples of good sources of protein. Many soybean products also contain all of the essential amino acids, but most plant proteins contain only some of the essential amino acids. However, you can combine plant proteins that complement each other to get all the amino acids that you need. Examples of plant proteins that complement each other are beans and rice or peanut butter and bread.

The amount of protein an adult needs depends on each person's size. You need 0.8 grams of protein per kilogram of body weight daily. (To calculate weight in kilograms, divide your weight in pounds by 2.2. For example, 130 pounds is equal to 59 kilograms.) A person who weighs 110 pounds (50 kilograms) needs approximately 40 grams of protein daily, whereas a person who weighs 198 pounds (90 kilograms) needs approximately 72 grams of protein daily. Women who are pregnant and lactating need 60 to 65 grams of protein per day. On the food label, calculations are based on a daily protein intake of 50 grams.

Most people in the United States consume more than the recommended amount of protein. The typical fast-food quarter-pound hamburger contains 28 grams of protein. Add cheese (5 grams) and a large order of fries, and you will have 39 grams of protein in one meal. Two beef burritos provide 44 grams. It is easy to see how most Americans consume sufficient protein. The average adult female takes in 65 grams of protein per day, and the average adult male consumes 105 grams of protein daily.

Many people choose to concentrate on plant rather than animal sources of proteins. Plant sources of proteins, such as beans and legumes, are usually low in fat and high in fiber. Combined with other plant sources that contain proteins, such as grains and vegetables, a plant-based diet can provide all of the necessary amino acids. In eastern Asian countries soy foods are a staple. The Japanese consume 10 to 50 grams of soy proteins per day compared to 1 to 3 grams daily in the United States.

In the past 10 years, more people in the United States have included soy proteins in their diets. In October 1999, the Food and Drug Administration authorized the use of a health claim on the food label for products containing at least 6.25 grams of soy protein per serving. The FDA acknowledged that 25 grams of soy protein a day as part of a diet low in saturated fat and cholesterol reduces the risk for heart disease. The FDA recommendation was based on the review of 38 studies. It should be pointed out that in most of the studies the soy proteins replaced the animal proteins in the diet. Only a few studies showed a benefit by adding soy proteins without reducing the amount of animal proteins. Soy products may confer other benefits, as explained in chapter 20.

How Am I Doing So Far?

Now let's go back to our original examples to see how to build a diet that provides a sufficient amount of protein. Anna weighs 130 pounds, so she needs approximately 47 grams of protein per day (130 pounds is equal to 59 kilograms; 59 kilograms × 0.8 grams of protein per kilogram = 47 grams of protein). She includes one egg at breakfast and adds cheese to her tortilla and beans at dinner. Her diet now contains 54 grams of protein, a sufficient amount. Notice that eggs and cheese do not contain fiber, and the egg adds just 1 gram of carbohydrate to the total. You will also notice that in the chart the word *carbohydrate* has been replaced with CHO, a common abbreviation based on the chemical makeup of carbohydrate (**C**arbon, **H**ydrogen, **O**xygen).

ANNA'S FOOD CHOICES: PROTEIN FOODS

Food	CHO (grams)	Fiber (grams)	Protein (grams)
2 slices whole-grain toast	24	4	6
1 poached egg	1	0	6
1 cup split pea soup (add water to dehydrated soup)	21	3	7
3½-inch bagel	38	2	7
Granola bar	19	1	2
2 flour tortillas	54	4	8
½ cup pinto beans	22	7	7
1½ oz cheddar cheese	0	0	10
15 tortilla chips	17	1	1
TOTAL SO FAR	196	22	54

Ellen adds a cup of milk at breakfast, cheese to her potato, and meat sauce to her spaghetti noodles. The meat sauce contains tomatoes that add carbohydrates and fiber. Any type of milk (nonfat or skim, 1%, 2%, low-fat, whole milk) is a source of carbohydrate as well as protein, but it contains no fiber.

ELLEN'S FOOD CHOICES: PROTEIN FOODS

Food	CHO (grams)	Fiber (grams)	Protein (grams)
1 cup instant oatmeal	36	4	8
1 cup nonfat milk	12	0	8
Baked potato with skin (approximately 7 oz)	51	5	5
2 oz American cheese	0	0	12
10 Dutch Twist pretzels	47	2	5
1 cup spaghetti noodles	40	4	7
1 cup canned tomato sauce with meat	37	8	8
2 slices French bread	26	2	4
1 cup microwave popcorn	4	1	1
TOTAL SO FAR	253	26	58

Ellen weighs 140 pounds and needs approximately 51 grams of protein daily (140 pounds is equal to 64 kilograms; 64 kilograms × 0.8 grams of protein per kilogram = 51 grams of protein). Her selection of foods so far provides enough protein to meet the recommendations.

Notice that each woman at this point is obtaining about the same amount of nutrients but from different foods. The combination of complex carbohydrates and protein foods reflects a pretty typical diet. But it is not a complete diet. Unfortunately for most Americans, one big category is lacking: fruits and vegetables.

Chapter 4

Fruits and Vegetables

For most people there is a simple way to improve their diets: Eat more fresh fruits and vegetables. Fresh fruits and vegetables provide carbohydrates, fiber, and vitamins as well as phytochemicals (compounds that are not nutrients but have biological activity). It is recommended that people consume **at least five fruits and vegetables per day**. Unfortunately, only about 25% of adults do. At least 75% of adults need to eat more fruits and vegetables daily.

Don't settle for poor-quality fruits and vegetables. The best fruits and vegetables are probably the ones that you or a neighbor grows in the backyard. They can be left on the tree or vine until they are fully ripe, and they are a real treat. The next-best choice is probably a roadside fruit stand or a farmer's market. Grocery stores provide the greatest variety, and the produce is often good, but sometimes the quality is disappointing. If you buy at the height of the season, fresh fruits and vegetables are high in quality and low in price.

Take-Home Message: In most cases, you can improve your diet by simply eating more fresh fruits and vegetables every day.

Consuming five fruits and vegetables a day is a good guideline. But there are substantial nutrient differences among fruits and vegetables, so you must choose carefully. Of those five, try to choose at least one that is a source of vitamin C and one that is a source of beta-carotene (a precursor to vitamin A) every day. Try to include cruciferous vegetables (see the following information) every other day.

Vitamin C is one of the antioxidants that can help protect your tissues from the harmful effects of oxygen. Eating vitamin C-containing foods daily may help prevent certain kinds of cancers and cardiovascular disease. Fruits and vegetables that are a source of beta-carotene protect you from breast and lung cancers and macular degeneration, a common form of blindness in older people.

Cruciferous vegetables are members of the cabbage family. Studies have shown that people who eat cruciferous vegetables regularly have a low rate of cancer compared to people who don't. The cabbage family consists of bok choy (Chinese white cabbage), broccoli, brussels sprouts, cabbage (both green and red), cauliflower, collard greens, kale, kohl-rabi, mustard greens, rutabagas, turnips, and turnip greens.

As you can see from the following chart, several of the cruciferous vegetables also contain vitamin C and beta-carotene. That means that they are packed full of nutrients thought to help prevent cancer. But you don't need to limit yourself to just cruciferous vegetables. Non-cruciferous vegetables are good too. In addition to the vitamin C and beta-carotene that may be present, all fruits and vegetables contain phytochemicals, compounds that are biologically active. Fruits and vegetables also contain carbohydrates and fiber. The bottom line is that you need to find a way to eat a variety of fruits and vegetables every day.

EXCEPTIONALLY NUTRITIOUS FRUITS AND VEGETABLES

Food	Vitamin C*	Beta-carotene*	Cruciferous*
Apricots		✔	
Blackberries	✔		
Bok choy	✔	✔	✔
Broccoli	✔	✔	✔
Brussels sprouts	✔		✔
Cabbage (red or green)	✔		✔
Cantaloupe	✔	✔	
Carrots		✔	
Cauliflower			✔
Chard		✔	
Collard greens		✔	✔
Grapefruit (whole or juice)	✔		
Honeydew melon	✔		
Kale	✔	✔	✔
Kiwi	✔		
Kohlrabi	✔		✔
Mango	✔	✔	
Mustard greens		✔	✔

EXCEPTIONALLY NUTRITIOUS FRUITS AND VEGETABLES (CONTINUED)

Food	Vitamin C*	Beta-carotene*	Cruciferous*
Orange (whole or juice)	✔		
Papaya	✔		
Peppers	✔	✔	
Pumpkin (fresh or canned)		✔	
Rutabaga	✔		✔
Snow peas	✔		
Spinach		✔	
Squash (acorn or butternut)		✔	
Strawberries	✔		
Sweet potatoes		✔	
Tomatoes	✔	✔	
Turnip	✔		✔
Turnip greens	✔	✔	✔

* To be included in the chart, a fruit or vegetable must contain at least 30 milligrams of vitamin C per serving, 225 micrograms retinol equivalents (RE) of vitamin A in the form of beta-carotene per serving, or be in the cruciferous family.

Importance of Vitamin C and Beta-Carotene

Many fruits and vegetables are excellent sources of vitamin C and beta-carotene. These two important vitamins will be the focus of this section. Both are antioxidants and may help protect your body from the effects of aging and chronic diseases such as some cancers and heart disease.

Oxygen is essential to life, so it may surprise you to learn that it can also destroy the body's tissues. Oxygen may undergo a chemical reaction in the body and become an unstable substance known as a free radical. Free radicals can destroy cellular membranes or DNA. The body has several systems to counteract the destructive effects of free radicals. One of these systems depends on the antioxidant vitamins: vitamin C, beta-carotene, and vitamin E. These vitamins react with the free radicals and keep them from destroying your cells. Daily servings of fruits and vegetables that contain vitamin C and beta-carotene provide your body with a ready supply of these antioxidants. Fruits and vegetables do contribute some vitamin E, but the best sources of vitamin E are vegetable oils and nuts. (Vitamin E will be discussed in chapter 7.)

Vitamins usually have more than one function in the body, and this is true for vitamin C and beta-carotene. Vitamin C is necessary for proper iron absorption. It also helps people resist infection, form scar tissue, and strengthen the walls of small blood vessels. Beta-carotene is converted to retinol (a form of vitamin A) in the body and is necessary for proper vision, healthy bones and teeth, and reproduction. These are important vitamins, so consuming the recommended amounts of each every day should be your goal. The Dietary Reference Intake (DRI) for vitamin C is 90 milligrams daily for adult men and 75 milligrams per day for adult women. Smoking destroys vitamin C, so men and women who smoke should consume 125 milligrams and 110 milligrams daily, respectively.

FABULOUS FOODS: VITAMIN C

The foods listed below contain at least 90 milligrams of vitamin C per serving; thus, each meets 100% or more of the daily requirement for adult, nonsmoking men and women.

1 cup (8 oz) orange juice or grapefruit juice

6 oz fresh broccoli (a small bunch)

1 medium red or yellow pepper (about 1/2 cup chopped)

1 medium hot green chili pepper

1/2 of a 5-inch cantaloupe

5 large strawberries

The amount of beta-carotene needed is not quite as easy to determine as the amount required for other vitamins. Studies have shown that people who eat fruits and vegetables containing beta-carotene have a lower risk for chronic disease, but scientists have not been able to measure exactly how much is necessary. The recommendation for vitamin A is based on total vitamin A intake, not just what is converted from beta-carotene. The Dietary Reference Intake for vitamin A is given in micrograms per day (mcg/day): 900 mcg/day for men and 700 mcg/day for women. Scientists emphasize that fruits and vegetables containing beta-carotene should be consumed daily as part of this recommended amount.

FABULOUS FOODS: BETA-CAROTENE

The foods listed below contain 100% or more of the daily requirement for Vitamin A for adults. The vitamin A is in the form of beta-carotene.

1 carrot (4 inches long)

1 cup raw kale (or equivalent cooked)

1/2 cup canned sweet potato (or the equivalent fresh)

3/4 cup cooked Butternut or Hubbard squash

3/4 cup cooked spinach (fresh or frozen)

1/2 cup carrot juice

1 cup cooked collard greens

Unfortunately for consumers, the amount of vitamin A in foods is reported in various ways. The DRI is stated in mcg (micrograms) of retinol equivalents (RE). However, older measures of vitamin A are still used, and sometimes you will see vitamin A reported as IU (international units). In fact, most supplements still use IU on the label. If you wish to convert the figures to compare them to the recommendations that are given in mcg, use the chart in appendix J. However, most consumers don't convert IU to mcg but look at the label to see the percentage of Daily Value that is met. This is an easy way to estimate whether you are getting a little (i.e., 10%) or a lot (i.e., 100%) without worrying about the actual amount.

Much emphasis has been placed on beta-carotene, but it is only one of several carotenoids (orange-colored pigments that occur naturally in fruits and vegetables). Other dietary carotenoids, such as lycopene and lutein, actually have stronger antioxidant activity than beta-carotene. Lycopene is found in tomatoes; lutein is found in green peas, spinach, and other green leafy vegetables. These foods provide a variety of carotenoids in the diet and several other compounds that exhibit antioxidant activity. Keep in mind that eating a variety of fruits and vegetables is an important goal.

Phytochemicals in Fruits, Vegetables, and Other Plant Foods

Phytochemicals are compounds that have biological activity, although they are not currently classified as nutrients. Our present knowledge of phytochemicals is very limited. There are thousands of phytochemicals in foods, and their identification and function are just being determined in many cases. Many phytochemicals are thought to help prevent cancer and cardiovascular disease. Scientists do not know the exact amount necessary to prevent disease or whether the phytochemicals work alone or in conjunction with other compounds. That is why the recommendation is to eat foods containing phytochemicals rather than to consume the phytochemical by itself. Anyone who says that an exact amount of a phytochemical will prevent a certain disease is probably trying to sell something. It is wise to include a variety of fruits, vegetables, and other plant foods in your diet and receive the benefits from the hundreds of phytochemicals in them. Three groups of phytochemicals are discussed here: *carotenoids, organosulfurs,* and *flavonoids.*

One large group of phytochemicals is carotenoids. At least 100 compounds are in the carotenoid group, including beta-carotene, which was discussed earlier. When you eat fruits and vegetables that are a good source of beta-carotene you also consume many other phytochemicals. The cruciferous vegetables contain several phytochemicals called indoles. All of the indoles appear to have anticancer properties, although each works in a different way.

Organosulfur compounds are phytochemicals found in onions, garlic, leeks, chives, and shallots. Animal studies have shown that the phytochemicals in these foods decrease the conversion of nitrate to nitrite in the gastrointestinal tract. Nitrite is known to be a cancer-causing compound. However, it is not known whether these phytochemicals have the same effect in the human gastrointestinal tract. If you like these foods, use them in your diet with the hope that these phytochemicals are beneficial. None of these foods is known to be harmful.

Of all the organosulfur compounds, garlic has received the most attention. At least 3,000 studies on garlic have been conducted. Scientists have been trying to determine the role that raw garlic plays in inhibiting bacterial growth in the stomach, preventing stomach or colon cancers, preventing heart disease, and stimulating the immune system. A daily intake of one to two cloves (approximately 4 grams) is often recommended, although more studies are required to determine the exact amount. The scientific evidence is stronger for the intake of raw or cooked garlic than it is for garlic supplements. Part II of this book contains more information on garlic and garlic supplements.

Another large group of phytochemicals is the flavonoids. This category contains about 4,000 compounds, including isoflavones, catechin, and theaflavins. Soybeans are the best-known source of isoflavones. Green tea contains catechin, and black tea contains theaflavins. These foods have received a lot of attention, but remember that many foods contain flavonoids, and more excellent sources will be identified in the future as a result of all the scientific research currently being conducted.

Because they are a concentrated source of isoflavones, soybeans have received a lot of attention. Soy products, with the exception of soy sauce, soybean oil, and soy lecithin, contain flavonoids such as isoflavones, compounds that are remarkably similar to estrogens in their chemical structure. In the United States, diets that do not include soybeans contain less than 1 milligram of isoflavones per day, a negligible amount. Traditional Japanese and Chinese diets, in which soybeans are a staple food, contain approximately 20 to 50 milligrams of isoflavones daily. Women who consume these traditional diets appear to have lower incidences of breast cancer, heart disease, and osteoporosis. However, it has not been determined whether the soy in the diet or other factors (low-fat, high-fiber diets and daily exercise) are major contributors to the reduced risk for these diseases. The usual advice prevails here: Obtain isoflavones from soy foods until more research is completed. Information on isoflavone supplements appears in chapter 20.

In addition to the flavonoids, plant foods may contain polyphenols. A subgroup of polyphenols is phenolic acids, compounds that are found in red wine, grapes, dark grape juice, and tea. These are not the only foods that contain phenolic acids, but they are concentrated sources. More information on tea and wine is found in chapter 9.

When scientific information is emerging but not yet confirmed, it is sometimes difficult to know what you should do while more research is being conducted. After all, the studies are promising. One approach is to consume more of the foods (but not excessive amounts) from the following chart.

SOME OF THE PHYTOCHEMICALS IN FOOD

Food	Carotenoids	Indoles	Organosulfur compounds	Flavonoids	Polyphenols
Dark orange fruits	✔				
Dark orange and green vegetables	✔				
Cruciferous vegetables		✔			
Onions, garlic, leeks, chives, shallots			✔		
Legumes (especially soybeans)				✔	
Green or black tea				✔	✔
Red wine, grapes, apples, oranges				✔	✔

How Am I Doing So Far?

Fruits and vegetables are not difficult to add to the diet. Anna figures that she needs something to drink with breakfast and that an easy way to get vitamin C is to drink fruit juice. She is willing to eat apples because they last longer than many fruits do. It never occurred to her that salsa is a good source of tomatoes, but she is glad that it is because she loves putting salsa on all kinds of foods. Anna likes the convenience of the small, peeled carrots that come in a bag.

Anna can consume an adequate amount of vitamin C and beta-carotene by including a few key foods in her diet. Just two foods, grapefruit juice and the tomato salsa, provide the daily recommended amount of vitamin C. Carrots are packed full of beta-carotene, so it is easy to obtain enough from just one simple food that needs no preparation. Anna includes a variety of plant foods in her diet, so she obtains phytochemicals from several sources as shown in the chart on the next page.

Ellen likes fruits and vegetables, but eating them routinely is a bit of a problem. She has noticed in the past that she'll get motivated to go to the store to purchase lots of fruits and vegetables. She has good intentions to make a salad for dinner but finds that she is too hungry and too tired once she gets home. She forgets to take the fruit to work. When it is time for her afternoon break, all that is available are vending machines with candy. By the end of the week the fruits and vegetables are no longer fresh or appealing, and she ends up throwing them out.

ANNA'S FOOD CHOICES: FRUITS AND VEGETABLES

Food	CHO (g)	Fiber (g)	Protein (g)	Vitamin C (mg)	Vitamin A (mcg RE)	Fruits or vegetables	Rich in phytochemicals
2 slices whole-grain toast	24	4	6	0	0		
1 poached egg	1	0	6	0	95		
1 cup grapefruit juice	22	0	1	72	2	2 servings	✓
1 cup black tea	0	0	0	0	0		✓
1 cup split pea soup (add water to dehydrated soup)	21	3	7	0	5		✓
3½-inch bagel	38	2	7	0	0		
3-inch apple	26	5	0	10	9	1 serving	
Granola bar	19	1	2	0	0		
2 flour tortillas	54	4	8	0	0		
½ cup pinto beans	22	7	7	2	0		✓
1½ oz cheddar cheese	0	0	10	0	127		
½ cup tomato salsa	8	0	0	40	176	1 serving	✓
15 tortilla chips	17	1	1	0	6		
4 small carrots	9	2.5	1	9	2531	1 serving	✓
TOTAL SO FAR	261	29.5	56	133	2951	5 servings	A variety of plant foods

ELLEN'S FOOD CHOICES: FRUITS AND VEGETABLES

Food	CHO (g)	Fiber (g)	Protein (g)	Vitamin C (mg)	Vitamin A (mcg RE)	Fruits or vegetables	Rich in phytochemicals
1 cup instant oatmeal	36	4	8	0	604		✔
1 cup nonfat milk	12	0	8	2	149		
1½-oz packet of raisins	33	3	0	0	0	1 serving	✔
Baked potato with skin (approximately 7 oz)	51	5	5	26	0		✔
2 oz American cheese	0	0	12	0	162		
Salad bar:						2 servings	
3 pieces Romaine lettuce	1	1	0	7	78		✔
8 cherry tomatoes	2	.5	0	8	28		✔
2 flowerets of cauliflower	1	.5	0	12	0		✔
4 red pepper strips	1	0	0	35	106		✔
8 oz orange juice	27	0	2	97	20	2 servings	✔
10 Dutch Twist pretzels	47	2	5	0	0		
1 cup spaghetti noodles	40	4	7	0	0		
1 cup canned tomato sauce with meat	37	8	8	26	577	1 serving	✔
2 slices French bread	26	2	4	0	0		
½ cup canned green beans	3	1	1	3	24	1 serving	✔
1 cup microwave popcorn	4	1	1	0	1		
TOTAL SO FAR	321	32	61	216	1749	7 servings	A variety of plant foods

The focus for Ellen needs to be easy foods: green salad at a salad bar, raisins, orange juice, and canned green beans would all fit the bill.

In this example, shown on the previous page, Ellen meets her daily vitamin C requirement with orange juice, but even without the orange juice she obtains a sufficient amount. Her salad provides more than 80% of her daily requirement. The tomatoes in the canned meat sauce gave her a large amount of beta-carotene. She ate seven servings of fruits and vegetables and obtained a variety of phytochemicals. Take note of the oatmeal in this example. Instant oatmeal is fortified with vitamin A and is a significant source in Ellen's diet. Oats do not naturally contain vitamin A, and most oats that are purchased are not fortified.

The nutrients in these sample diets come from a variety of carbohydrates, protein foods, and fruits and vegetables. Next, we'll add calcium-containing foods.

Chapter 5

Calcium Foods

Calcium, a mineral, is associated with bone health. This is not surprising because 99% of the calcium in your body is in the bones. But it is the other 1%, found mainly in your blood that dictates things. The calcium in your blood is used for muscle contraction, nerve impulse transmission, blood clotting, and regulation of blood pressure. These important functions cannot be left to chance, so your body strictly maintains the amount of calcium in your blood. What supplies the calcium in your blood? The calcium you consume from food or calcium supplements and the calcium that is stored in your bones.

> *Take-Home Message: Everyone needs calcium every day. Milk is an excellent source, but not the only source, of calcium.*

Calcium is found in a variety of food sources. One of the best known is cow's milk. An 8-ounce glass contains about 300 milligrams. Other dairy products, such as 1¹/₂ ounces of cheddar cheese, contain the same amount as milk. But some people don't like milk or dairy products, and many adults are lactose intolerant. They must find a way to get enough calcium from other sources.

Obtaining calcium from nondairy sources is difficult for many people because the amount of calcium in vegetables is low. For example, 1 cup of cooked broccoli has about 100 milligrams of calcium, one-third of the calcium that milk does. Additionally, good vegetable sources of calcium (brussels sprouts, collard greens, green cabbage, kale, kohlrabi, mustard greens, turnip greens) are not everyday foods for many Americans.

FABULOUS FOODS: CALCIUM

The foods listed below contain at least 300 milligrams of calcium per serving thus each meets approximately 30% of the daily requirement for adults ages 19-50.

1 cup milk	**1¹/₂ cup cooked turnip greens**
1 cup buttermilk	**1 can (85 grams) sardines**
1 cup yogurt	**1 cup calcium-fortified orange juice**
1 cup calcium-fortified soy milk	

People all over the world obtain calcium from a variety of sources. Sardines and other small fish eaten whole provide calcium because the fish bones are an excellent source. Tofu that has been preserved with calcium and some seaweed are also good calcium sources. Mineral water, depending on the brand, may provide 50 milligrams of calcium in an 8-ounce glass. The bottom line is that you need calcium and there are many ways to obtain the calcium that you need. The following chart shows many strategies for getting the required amount of calcium. Choose those that feel right for you.

STRATEGIES FOR GETTING ENOUGH CALCIUM

Drink milk and milk products.
Drink milk and milk products but use lactase tablets or consume lactase-treated products.
Consume fermented milk products such as yogurt and aged cheese.
Consume nondairy calcium foods such as cabbage, broccoli, turnips, and other greens.
Consume calcium-fortified products such as orange juice, soy milk, and cereal (check labels).
Consume calcium supplements.

The calcium recommendation for adults is based on age. Those aged 19 to 50 need to consume 1,000 milligrams per day. After age 50, 1,200 milligrams of calcium daily is needed. Postmenopausal women not receiving estrogen (hormone replacement therapy) should consume 1,500 milligrams per day. Meeting calcium requirements is important for all adults. Consuming 1,000 to 1,200 milligrams daily is easier for men than for women. Most men consume more food and therefore more calcium than women do. Obtaining 1,500 milligrams from diet alone is difficult. Calcium supplements are a reasonable alternative for some people and are covered in chapter 19.

How Am I Doing So Far?

Anna is 26 years old, so she needs 1,000 milligrams of calcium every day. Anna doesn't drink milk, so she thought that her diet wouldn't have much calcium. But the cheese is a big contributor, and the tortillas provide some calcium too. Two scoops of her favorite low-fat frozen yogurt help her meet her calcium requirement. Anna consumes enough dairy products to meet the requirement even though she is not a milk drinker.

ANNA'S FOOD CHOICES: CALCIUM-CONTAINING FOODS

Food	CHO (g)	Fiber (g)	Protein (g)	Vitamin C (mg)	Vitamin A (mcg RE)	Calcium (mg)
2 slices whole-grain toast	24	4	6	0	0	48
1 poached egg	1	0	6	0	95	24
1 cup grapefruit juice	22	0	1	72	2	17
1 cup black tea	0	0	0	0	0	0
1 cup split pea soup (add water to dehydrated soup)	21	3	7	0	5	20
3½-inch bagel	38	2	7	0	0	52
3-inch apple	26	5	0	10	9	12
Granola bar	19	1	2	0	0	29
2 flour tortillas	54	4	8	0	0	122
½ cup pinto beans	22	7	7	2	0	41
1½ oz cheddar cheese	0	0	10	0	127	303
½ cup tomato salsa	8	0	0	40	176	8
15 tortilla chips	17	1	1	0	6	42
4 small carrots	9	2.5	1	9	2531	24
2 scoops (slightly more than a cup) low-fat frozen yogurt	30	0	8	2	2	274
TOTAL SO FAR	291	29.5	64	135	2953	1016

Ellen likes milk and cheese, which are the main sources of calcium in her diet. The instant oatmeal is a significant source too. Along with vitamin A, instant oatmeal has calcium added; oatmeal in the box (regular or quick oats) does not. Both Anna and Ellen can meet their calcium requirements through diet alone but only because they consume milk or milk products.

ELLEN'S FOOD CHOICES:
CALCIUM-CONTAINING FOODS

Food	CHO (g)	Fiber (g)	Protein (g)	Vitamin C (mg)	Vitamin A (mcg RE)	Calcium (mg)
1 cup instant oatmeal	36	4	8	0	604	218
1 cup nonfat milk	12	0	8	2	149	301
1½-oz packet of raisins	33	3	0	0	0	21
Baked potato with skin (approximately 7 oz)	51	5	5	26	0	20
2 oz American cheese	0	0	12	0	162	344
Salad bar:						
3 pieces Romaine lettuce	1	1	0	7	78	11
8 cherry tomatoes	2	.5	0	8	28	2
2 flowerets of cauliflower	1	.5	0	12	0	6
4 red pepper strips	1	0	0	35	106	2
8 oz orange juice	27	0	2	97	20	22
10 Dutch Twist pretzels	47	2	5	0	0	22
1 cup spaghetti noodles	40	4	7	0	0	10
1 cup canned meat sauce	37	8	8	26	577	68
2 slices French bread	26	2	4	0	0	38
½ cup canned green beans	3	1	1	3	24	18
1 cup microwave popcorn	4	1	1	0	1	0
TOTAL SO FAR	321	32	61	216	1749	1103

Getting Calcium From Nondairy Sources

Both Anna and Ellen include dairy products in their diets and met their calcium requirements, but many people do not want to consume dairy products. The following chart shows how you could obtain 1,000 milligrams of calcium from nondairy sources. (Note that this diet focuses on calcium only and is not complete.)

OBTAINING CALCIUM FROM NONDAIRY SOURCES

Food	Calcium (mg)
2 pancakes	176
1 cup blackberries	46
1 whole-wheat English muffin	175
2 tablespoons peanut butter	12
2 figs	54
8 oz San Pellegrino mineral water	50
4 oz canned salmon	240

OBTAINING CALCIUM FROM NONDAIRY SOURCES
(CONTINUED)

Food	Calcium (mg)
1 cup broccoli	94
1 oz almonds	74
½ cup cooked acorn squash	54
1 mixed grain roll	24
1 medium orange	52
TOTAL CALCIUM	1051

The diets we're building comprise nutrients from carbohydrates, protein foods, fruits and vegetables, and calcium-containing foods. Calcium isn't the only mineral your body needs. Iron-containing foods are another essential part of a healthy diet.

Chapter 6

Iron Foods

Iron, a mineral, is associated with healthy blood. The recommended daily intake of iron is 8 milligrams for men and for women who have been through menopause. Premenopausal women lose iron in blood when they menstruate, so they have a much higher need for iron— 18 milligrams daily. Consuming 8 milligrams of iron each day is easy, especially for men. Obtaining 18 milligrams of dietary iron is difficult, and many women of childbearing age have an iron deficiency. Women who are pregnant are routinely prescribed a multivitamin and mineral supplement containing sufficient iron to meet the demands of pregnancy.

Although there are some excellent sources of iron (3 ounces of steamed clams contain almost 27 milligrams), iron is usually gathered from a variety of foods. The small amount of iron found in any one food may not appear to be much; but when all the small amounts are added together, the daily requirement can be met. Most likely you will gather a small amount from a variety of foods (meat, fish, poultry, dried beans, breads, fruits, and vegetables).

Iron absorbed from foods is used to replenish iron stores and provide iron for red blood cells. If you do not consume enough iron in your diet you are at risk for iron-deficiency anemia because iron stores will be used up and not replenished. Eventually the red blood cells will be smaller and contain less iron, and you will feel tired and fatigued.

At risk is a commonly used medical term. Certain factors are associated with disease but by themselves do not predict that you will get the disease. Cigarette smoking is a risk factor for lung cancer, and the majority of people who have lung cancer smoke cigarettes. However, some people who smoke do not get lung cancer, and a few people who have never smoked also get lung cancer. But if you look at the big picture, cigarette smoking puts you at risk for developing lung cancer. In the same way, lack of iron in the diet is associated with iron-deficiency anemia. Many people who consume too little iron have this disease. However, not all people who consume less than the recommended amount of iron will develop iron-deficiency anemia. This can be explained by individual differences in the way people absorb iron. The following chart is a list of iron-containing foods.

IRON-CONTAINING FOODS

Food	Iron (mg)
3 oz steamed clams	26.6
5 steamed oysters	5-16.5
1 cup cereal (iron added; depends on the brand)	2-16
3 oz beef liver	5.3
3 oz beef	3
1 cup tuna fish	2.4
¹/₂ cup pinto beans	2.09
3 oz chicken (dark meat has more)	1.5
¹/₂ cup spinach, cooked from frozen (fresh spinach that is cooked has twice as much)	1.44
1 cup soy milk	1.42
¹/₂ cup tofu	1.3
1¹/₂ oz raisins	.87
1 slice bread (iron added; amount varies based on the kind of bread)	.80
1 egg, white and yolk	.72

A person with particularly good iron absorption may take in less than the recommended amount but won't have iron-deficiency anemia because she absorbs a high proportion of the iron she consumes. Because it is difficult to know how well you absorb iron, the best strategy is to consume the recommended amount of iron daily.

FABULOUS FOODS: IRON

The foods listed below contain a substantial amount of iron, 4 to 16 milligrams per serving. Men and postmenopausal women need 8 milligrams daily and menstruating women need 18 milligrams daily.

1 cup canned chili and beans (8 mg of iron)

1 can (about 1.5 oz) oysters (6 mg of iron)

2 1/2 tablespoons hijiki seaweed (5.5 mg of iron)

1 cup iron fortified instant oatmeal or cream of wheat (10 mg of iron)

1 cup iron fortified ready to eat breakfast cereal (6 to 16 mg of iron)

How Am I Doing So Far?

Anna is 26 years old and needs 18 milligrams of iron daily. Her dietary intake is about 15 milligrams. Her intake puts her at risk for iron-deficiency anemia, but it does not mean that she has iron-deficiency anemia. Her physician would be able to determine whether she has iron-deficiency anemia by looking at the results of a blood test for hemoglobin. Her dietary intake is about 15 milligrams (see chart on page 50).

Ellen was able to meet the recommended level of iron intake through her diet but only because she ate an iron-fortified food. Her two packets of instant oatmeal provided an exceptional source of iron (8.4 milligrams). The manufacturer added the iron to the oatmeal (the equivalent amount of regular or quick oats contains only 1.59 milligrams). If Ellen had not eaten instant oatmeal, she would have consumed 13.27 milligrams of iron, below the recommendation for a woman of childbearing age. Ellen's sample diet so far is shown on page 51.

The sample diets now include quite a variety of foods. Some of these foods, such as fabulous foods, are nutrient-rich. Other foods may be surprising sources of nutrients. Remember the discussion of "Should I not . . ."? Many people ask, "Should I not eat fat?" Let's turn our attention to the role of fats and fat-soluble vitamins.

ANNA'S FOOD CHOICES: IRON-CONTAINING FOODS

Food	CHO (g)	Fiber (g)	Protein (g)	Vitamin C (mg)	Vitamin A (mcg RE)	Calcium (mg)	Iron (mg)
2 slices whole-grain toast	24	4	6	0	0	48	1.8
1 poached egg	1	0	6	0	95	24	.72
1 cup grapefruit juice	22	0	1	72	2	17	.49
1 cup black tea	0	0	0	0	0	0	.05
1 cup split pea soup (add water to dehydrated soup)	21	3	7	0	5	20	.94
3½-inch bagel	38	2	7	0	0	52	2.53
3-inch apple	26	5	0	10	9	12	.32
Granola bar	19	1	2	0	0	29	.72
2 flour tortillas	54	4	8	0	0	122	3.24
½ cup pinto beans	22	7	7	2	0	41	2.22
1½ oz cheddar cheese	0	0	10	0	127	303	.28
½ cup tomato salsa	8	0	0	40	176	8	.48
15 tortilla chips	17	1	1	0	6	42	.4
4 small carrots	9	2.5	1	9	2531	24	.45
2 scoops (slightly more than a cup) low-fat frozen yogurt	30	0	8	2	2	274	.14
TOTAL SO FAR	291	29.5	64	135	2953	1016	14.78

ELLEN'S FOOD CHOICES: IRON-CONTAINING FOODS

Food	CHO (g)	Fiber (g)	Protein (g)	Vitamin C (mg)	Vitamin A (mcg RE)	Calcium (mg)	Iron (mg)
1 cup instant oatmeal	36	4	8	0	604	218	8.4
1 cup nonfat milk	12	0	8	2	149	301	.1
1½-oz packet of raisins	33	3	0	0	0	21	.87
Baked potato with skin (approximately 7 oz)	51	5	5	26	0	20	2.75
2 oz American cheese	0	0	12	0	162	344	.22
Salad bar:							
3 pieces Romaine lettuce	1	1	0	7	78	11	.33
8 cherry tomatoes	2	.5	0	8	28	2	.20
2 flowerets of cauliflower	1	.5	0	12	0	6	.11
4 red pepper strips	1	0	0	35	106	2	.08
8 oz orange juice	27	0	2	97	20	22	.25
10 Dutch Twist pretzels	47	2	5	0	0	22	2.59
1 cup spaghetti noodles	40	4	7	0	0	10	1.96
1 cup canned meat sauce	37	8	8	26	577	68	1.94
2 slices French bread	26	2	4	0	0	38	1.26
½ cup canned green beans	3	1	1	3	24	18	.61
1 cup microwave popcorn	4	1	1	0	1	0	.14
TOTAL SO FAR	321	32	61	216	1749	1103	21.81

Chapter 7

Fats and Fat-Soluble Vitamins

In a weight-loss-crazy society, undue attention may be given to the amount of fat in the diet. Because fat contains more calories per gram (approximately 9) than any other nutrient (carbohydrates and proteins contain 4 calories per gram, and alcohol contains 7 calories per gram), it is a major focus for many weight-loss diets. But this book is written from a different perspective: to know the nutrients that you need and the foods that contain those nutrients. Experts agree that everyone needs fat in their diet.

Fats are made up of long chains of fatty acids. The body can make most, but not all, of the fatty acids it needs. Those that it cannot make are called essential fatty acids, and they must be consumed in the diet. One reason that you must have fat in your diet is to provide these essential fatty acids. Another reason to consume dietary fat is that fat carries the fat-soluble vitamins needed by your body. Vitamins A, D, E, and K are transported by fat, and the fat helps them to be absorbed. Specific information about each of these vitamins is given in the following section.

As odd as it may sound, fat needs to be consumed *because* it provides calories. Fat is a concentrated energy (calorie) source, and it would be difficult to meet your energy needs with just carbohydrates and proteins. That said, your need for fat is not unlimited. Determining just how much dietary fat healthy people need is a difficult task.

Since the 1970s a consistent public health message has been to reduce dietary fat intake. This message is based on studies that show that saturated fats (found in animal fats such as meat and dairy products) increase blood cholesterol, which in turn increases the risk of heart attack in people with heart disease. But this book is not written for people who have been diagnosed with heart disease. The evidence that consuming a low-fat diet will reduce the risk of heart disease for people without heart disease is not very compelling. Scientific studies show a weak correlation between reducing dietary fat intake and a decreased risk of heart disease in healthy people.

Scientists continue to study the issue of how much dietary fat people need. A frequent recommendation has been to consume 30% or less of total daily calories as dietary fat. If your diet contains 2,000 calories, then the recommended intake of fat would be 67 grams or less per day. (The formula is as follows: 2,000 calories multiplied by 30% equals 600 calories from fat. Thus, 600 calories from fat divided by 9 calories per gram of fat equals 67 grams of fat.) The newest recommendation suggests 20 to 35 % of total calories from fat as an acceptable range. Try to get much of this fat from fish, nuts, seeds, and vegetable oils.

Take-Home Message: Fish, nuts, seeds, and vegetable oils are the preferred sources of fat.

Although a low-fat diet may not reduce heart disease risk for healthy people, certain kinds of dietary fats may protect against heart disease and are associated with good health. These fats include omega-3 fatty acids (found in fish and seed oils), monounsaturated fats (found in nuts and olive oil), and polyunsaturated fats (found in vegetable oils).

When oils are hardened, the process, called hydrogenation, changes the structure and the health benefits of the vegetable and nut oils. Most baked goods and snack foods contain hydrogenated oils, as do most margarines and peanut butter. Hydrogenation produces trans fatty acids, a type of fatty acid that tends to raise blood cholesterol levels. Trans fatty acids provide no health benefits, so consumption should be as low as possible (completely avoiding trans fatty acids would be very difficult). As you would with whole grains, choose fat-containing foods that have been minimally processed.

One of the benefits of consuming fat is the intake of the fat-soluble vitamins—vitamins A, D, E, and K. Vitamin A is found as preformed vitamin A (retinol) in animal foods (such as milk) or as a vitamin A pre-cursor (beta-carotene) in orange and dark green vegetables. Beta-carotene can be converted to retinol, which is used by many cells and tissues throughout your body. As discussed previously, beta-carotene, but not retinol, acts as an antioxidant, which protects cells from the damaging effects of oxygen and lowers your risk for heart disease and diet-related cancers. Some studies show that a diet rich in beta-carotene is correlated with a low rate of macular degeneration, one form of blindness that accompanies old age.

Vitamin D is not easily categorized. It is a fat-soluble vitamin, but it is also a hormone (regulator). It is found in food, but it is also converted from ultraviolet light (UV). People can suffer from a deficiency (if they don't have exposure to sunlight or vitamin D-containing foods) or from a toxicity (caused by oversupplementation). Light-skinned people can convert a day's worth of vitamin D from 15 minutes of exposure to ultraviolet light, whereas dark-skinned people need about 3 hours of sunlight to convert a sufficient amount. The body regulates the amount converted so there is no danger of vitamin D toxicity caused by UV exposure. The recommended intake of vitamin D for adults is based on age. In the absence of sufficient ultraviolet light exposure, adults up to age 50 need 5 micrograms (mcg) daily. Those 51 to 70 years of age need 10 micrograms daily, and those over age 70 need 15 micrograms per day. The increased requirements reflect your body's decreased vitamin D activity, a result of the aging process.

Vitamin E is also a powerful antioxidant. Much of the vitamin E research has been conducted on the lungs and the red blood cells because those cells have constant exposure to oxygen. Athletes are particularly interested in the benefits of vitamin E because of the role it might play in protecting muscle tissue from oxygen damage. There may also be a connection between vitamin E and heart disease as studies have shown that men who have the lowest vitamin E intake have more heart attacks than men who have higher vitamin E consumption. Vitamin E, in conjunction with vitamin C, appears to protect arteries from oxygen damage.

The recommended vitamin E intake for adults is 15 milligrams per day of alpha-tocopherol. Alpha-tocopherol is a biologically active form of vitamin E found naturally in food. Three forms of synthetic vitamin E are thought to have the same biological activity as alpha-tocopherol. Although vitamin E is assumed to protect against heart disease and possibly other chronic disease, the evidence is not yet strong enough to recommend a level of intake greater than 15 milligrams per day for the general public. Vitamin E has the lowest toxicity of the fat-soluble vitamins, and the tolerable upper intake level is set at 1,000 milligrams (an amount that can be obtained only through supplements).

FABULOUS FOODS: VITAMIN E

The foods listed below contain at least 6 milligrams of vitamin E per serving; thus, each meets 40% or more of the daily requirement for adults.

1 tablespoon safflower oil	1 oz almonds
1 tablespoon sunflower oil	1 oz hazelnuts
3 tablespoons peanut butter	1/4 cup sunflower seeds

Vitamin K is not mentioned as frequently as the other fat-soluble vitamins because deficiencies are rare. People obtain vitamin K from foods, notably green leafy vegetables. Bacteria living in the gastrointestinal tract provide at least half of the vitamin K. People who lack the bacteria to synthesize vitamin K obtain the necessary amount needed only by prescription because supplemental vitamin K is potentially toxic.

How Am I Doing So Far?

Let's take another look at Anna's diet. So far she has built a diet containing 291 grams of carbohydrate, 64 grams of protein, and 41 grams of fat. She has nearly met the recommended carbohydrate goal and has exceeded the goal for protein. At this point, Anna has consumed about two-thirds of the fat recommended (assuming she takes in 2,000 calories daily).

Anna adds more fat to her diet. The source of the fat is nuts—peanut butter and almonds. Notice the amounts of vitamin E and fiber 1 ounce of almonds contributes. Also notice that the nuts provide some carbohydrates and that she has now met her goals for all three macronutrients—carbohydrate, protein, and fat.

ANNA'S FOOD CHOICES:
FAT- AND VITAMIN E-CONTAINING FOODS

Food	CHO (g)	Fiber (g)	Protein (g)	Fat (g)	Vitamin E (mg)
2 slices whole-grain toast	24	4	6	2	.32
1 poached egg	1	0	6	5	.52
1 cup grapefruit juice	22	0	1	<1	.12
1 cup black tea	0	0	0	0	0
1 cup split pea soup (add water to dehydrated soup)	21	3	7	1	.13
3½-inch bagel	38	2	7	1	.02
1 tablespoon peanut butter	3	1	4	8	1.6
3-inch apple	26	5	0	<1	.56
Granola bar	19	1	2	5	.34
2 flour tortillas	54	4	8	6	1.24
½ cup pinto beans	22	7	7	<1	.8
1½ oz cheddar cheese	0	0	10	13	.15
½ cup tomato salsa	8	0	0	<1	.32
15 tortilla chips	17	1	1	8	.36
4 small carrots	9	2.5	1	<1	.41
2 scoops (slightly more than a cup) low-fat frozen yogurt	30	0	8	<1	<.01
1 oz almonds	6	3	6	15	6.72
TOTAL SO FAR	300	33.5	74	64	13.61

Anna's fat intake is 64 grams, a very appropriate amount. Her intake of vitamin E falls just short of the 15 milligrams recommended daily. This is not cause for concern because vitamin E is a fat-soluble vitamin and can be stored in the body. Diets vary from day to day, and it is likely that some days she consumes more vitamin E and some days she would consume less. Vitamin E is a popular supplement because meeting vitamin E requirements through diet alone is not always easy (see chapter 19 for more information on vitamin E supplements). In Anna's case, if she did not include almonds she would fall far short of the recommended levels of vitamin E.

Ellen adds nuts and seeds to her diet, both of which are excellent sources of vitamin E and fiber. A natural addition to her salad is dressing made with vegetable oil, also a good source of vitamin E.

ELLEN'S FOOD CHOICES:
FAT- AND VITAMIN E-CONTAINING FOODS

Food	CHO (g)	Fiber (g)	Protein (g)	Fat (g)	Vitamin E (mg)
1 cup instant oatmeal	36	4	8	2	.28
1 cup nonfat milk	12	0	8	<1	.1
1½-oz packet of raisins	33	3	0	<1	.3
Baked potato with skin (approximately 7 oz)	51	5	5	<1	.1
2 oz American cheese	0	0	12	18	.26
Salad bar:					
3 pieces Romaine lettuce	1	1	0	<1	.13
8 cherry tomatoes	2	.5	0	<1	.17
2 flowerets of cauliflower	1	.5	0	<1	.01
4 red pepper strips	1	0	0	<1	.13
1 tablespoon sunflower seeds	2	1	2	5	4.52
1 tablespoon Italian dressing	2	0	<1	7	1.56
8 oz orange juice	27	0	2	<1	.47
10 Dutch Twist pretzels	47	2	5	2	.13
1 cup spaghetti noodles	40	4	7	1	.08
1 cup canned meat sauce	37	8	8	14	5.91
2 slices French bread	26	2	4	2	.12
½ cup canned green beans	3	1	1	<1	.09
1 cup microwave popcorn	4	1	1	1	.06
1 oz pistachios	7	3	6	14	1.46
TOTAL SO FAR	332	36	69	66	15.88

Ellen's fat and vitamin E intakes are within the recommended ranges. Although she includes animal fats in her diet (cheese and meat in the spaghetti sauce), half of her fat comes from nuts, seeds, and vegetable oil.

The sample diets, each representing just one day's worth of nutrients, include whole-grain carbohydrates, protein foods, fruits and vegetables, vitamins, minerals, and fats. The goal is to meet your body's nutrient needs without exceeding your body's caloric needs. So you need to balance nutrient intake with caloric intake to maintain a healthy body weight. In chapter 8 you will find a discussion of energy (caloric) needs.

Chapter 8

Consuming Enough Energy

By now you should be convinced that diet is a pattern of eating, not a weight-loss plan. After all, this chapter devoted to energy and the measure of energy—calories—isn't the first chapter! Energy intake is an important element in diet planning, but it should not be the sole focus of your diet.

Your body needs energy to do work. Energy is in foods containing carbohydrates, fats, proteins, and alcohol. You need to eat to provide enough energy for your body. (Energy is measured in Calories or kilocalories [the scientifically correct term], but the lower-cased term *calorie* is often used in the United States; thus, we use that term in this book.)

To illustrate how twisted things have gotten in a weight-loss-diet crazy society, consider the following analogy. Your body is a car. You need to put gallons of fuel in the car to run it. Most people refer to the gallons as ounces. People would constantly worry that their cars had too many ounces of fuel that day. Sounds silly, doesn't it?

Your body is not a car, but there are some similarities between your body and a car. Both need energy to do work. Your body gets energy from food, and your car gets its energy from gasoline. When you are hungry you need more fuel, just as the car needs more fuel when the gas gauge is low. An important concept in human nutrition is the need to consume enough food to provide fuel for the body to perform work.

But bodies and cars are different when it comes to excess fuel intake. You can consume more energy (calories) than you need for performing the work that you do. The excess energy is stored as body fat, and there is little physical limitation to storing more fat. Cars, on the other hand, have a predetermined limit to their fuel storage;

the size of the gas tank dictates how much fuel it can store. If your car were like your body, excess gasoline would be pumped into the seats and the tires and could be used later.

At this point the important question is this: "How much energy is needed to provide the fuel for the body's work?" The answer depends on your gender and how much physical activity you perform. The exact number of calories cannot be predicted, but the following guidelines give a reasonable estimate.

APPROXIMATE DAILY ENERGY NEEDS

	Sedentary males and sedentary nonpregnant females	Active males and active nonpregnant females
Energy/day	14 calories per pound of body weight	15 to 17 calories per pound of body weight

Anytime a complicated concept is reduced to a simple chart, there are always problems. This chart is based on body weight, but energy needs are more accurately predicted when based on body composition (the amount of muscle tissue and the amount of body fat). If you are active and have more muscle than most people of your weight, use the higher end of the guideline (17 calories per pound of body weight) to estimate your daily energy needs. If you engage in athletic training and have a lot of muscle, these estimates are too low.

Another problem is the use of current body weight. If current body weight is high because of excess body fat, then using this guideline may result in an estimated energy intake that is too high. For example, using this formula, a 250-pound sedentary female would estimate that she needs 3,500 calories per day (250 pounds multiplied by 14 calories per pound). In reality, 3,500 calories per day would probably be too much for maintaining weight. It may be more realistic for a woman of this weight to estimate her intake at 2,000 calories per day. Males whose current weight is high because of excess body fat could estimate their intake at 2,500 calories per day.

The caloric guideline is based on the energy needed to maintain current body weight. But is your current weight a healthy weight? Does your current weight put you at a greater risk for disease? Unfortunately, these are not easy questions to answer.

Healthy Body Weight

Let's define a healthy body weight as one that decreases the risk of disease and premature death. It is not based on appearance. Overall, weight is a crude (imprecise) measure and not an accurate predictor of health for a given person. But it is a convenient measure because most people have access to a scale. And there is an association between increasing weight and increasing risk of disease, although this is not true for all people.

Body mass index (BMI), which measures the relationship between height and weight, is a widely used guideline to determine a healthy body weight. The BMI formula assumes that adult height is stable and that any increase in scale weight is a result of an increase in body fat. BMI should not be used with pregnant females (whose increase in weight is due to more muscle, blood, and fluid as well as fat) or trained athletes (whose increase in weight is mostly due to increased muscle). BMI is not accurate for people who have decreased in height because of osteoporosis.

If you are a Caucasian adult under age 65 who is not pregnant and not a trained athlete, a BMI of 25 or more is associated with an increased risk for disease. (The unit of measure of BMI is kg/m^2 although the unit of measure often does not appear.) Note that most of the studies have been conducted on young or middle-aged Caucasian (white) populations, and it is not known whether the association holds true for other populations. In adults over age 65, a BMI of 30 or more is associated with increased disease risk. You can calculate your BMI using the following formula or by checking the chart in appendix K. Keep in mind that height is measured without shoes and weight is measured without clothes.

HOW TO CALCULATE BODY MASS INDEX

$$BMI = weight\ (kg) \div height^2\ (meters)$$

Step 1. Convert body weight from pounds to kilograms by dividing weight in pounds by 2.2 kilograms per pound. For example, 110 pounds = 50 kilograms.

Step 2. Convert height in inches to meters by multiplying height in inches by .0254 meters per inch. For example, 64 inches (5'4") = 1.63 meters.

Step 3. Weight (kilograms) $\div$ by $height^2$ (meters) = 50 kilograms $\div (1.63)^2$ = 18.8.

A BMI between 18.5 and 25 is considered a healthy body weight for adults under the age of 65. However, this general guideline needs further examination. A person may have a low body weight caused by smoking. Smokers, on average, weigh less but die sooner than non-smokers. A person with a low body weight may also have a disease (in some cases undiagnosed) that results in a low weight. Disordered eating patterns, such as anorexia and bulimia, may result in low body weight but poor nutrient status. If your weight is low for any of these reasons, your risk for disease and premature death is increased even though your BMI falls in the healthy body weight range. There are also disease risks associated with a BMI less than 18.5, a clear case where less is not better.

What does it mean if your BMI is greater than 25 (or greater than 30 if over the age of 65)? It means that the risk for certain diseases is greater, but it does not mean that you will necessarily have those diseases. In women, as BMI increases from 30 to above 35 (obese) and then above 40 (extremely obese), there is a greater risk for high blood pressure, gallbladder disease, type 2 (adult-onset) diabetes, heart disease, and osteoarthritis. This is not true for every woman, but as a general statement it is true for women as a group.

If your current BMI is above 25 (or 30 if you are older), your risk for these diseases is greater than for a woman whose BMI is less than 25. However, if you look at individuals within the group, some will not reflect the general trend. For example, the majority of women who have a BMI greater than 40 will have one or more of the diseases mentioned; but there will be women with a BMI greater than 40 who have none of the diseases mentioned even though they are categorized as extremely obese. In every BMI category there will be women with normal blood pressure, normal blood glucose (sugar), and normal blood lipid (fat) levels. Weight alone is not a predictor of disease.

In men, the trends are not as clear. The strongest association is between increasing BMI and high blood pressure. The risk for osteoarthritis and gallbladder disease does increase as BMI increases above 25 (or 30 for those over the age of 65), but neither of these diseases is as prevalent in obese males as they are in obese females. The risk for high blood cholesterol is actually greater for men with a BMI between 30 and 35 than for men with a BMI greater than 40.

It is also important to remember that having a BMI of less than 25 does not mean that your risk of disease is zero. For men and women who are in the "healthiest" BMI category, 23% have high blood pressure and 27% have high blood cholesterol. The bottom line is that BMI may be a useful guideline, but it is only that—a guideline. Each person must find out more specific information by having blood pressure, blood glucose, and blood lipids (cholesterol, triglycerides, and other types of fats) measured.

Take-Home Message: Body weight is an imprecise measure of health. For many people, getting fatter means an increased chance of having high blood pressure, diabetes, and other diseases. See your doctor to find out whether you have these diseases.

Another healthy weight issue is weight stability. It is recommended that nonpregnant adults over the age of 21 should not gain more than 10 pounds as they age. It is assumed that this 10-pound weight gain is fat, not muscle. Two large studies have shown that people who gain less than 10 pounds as they age (considered weight stable) are at a lower risk for disease than those who gained 11 to 22 pounds. Those who gained more than 22 pounds as they aged were at the greatest risk. The diseases where risk was increased were heart disease, adult-onset diabetes, high blood pressure, and gallstones.

If you are over the age of 50, be aware that as you age muscle mass tends to decrease and that fat, especially abdominal fat, tends to increase. In many older people body weight is stable but their body shape is changing, and they find that they are getting rounder around the waist. If fat is accumulating in the abdominal cavity and is surrounding the organs, then your risk for diabetes and heart disease is increased. The fat stored in the abdominal area is very mobile, and the easy transport of abdominal fat into the blood-stream increases the risk for these diseases.

Remember that body weight is an imprecise predictor of health. It is much better to focus on more precise measures such as blood pressure, blood tests, and measures of fitness. Some ways to measure fitness include aerobic (heart and lung) endurance, muscular strength, muscular endurance, and flexibility. Unfortunately, some of these are difficult or impossible for people to measure by themselves.

How Am I Doing So far?

Anna is 5'6" tall, weighs 130 pounds, and falls into the sedentary category. People are considered sedentary if they do little physical activity throughout the day. On a normal day Anna gets ready for work, drives for 30 minutes, works at a desk job, drives home, fixes dinner, reads, and watches television. By using the guideline (130 pounds × 14 calories per pound), Anna calculates that she needs approximately 1,820 calories per day. The diet that Anna has been building contains approximately 2,120 calories as shown in the following table. If her energy output is approximately 1,820 calories daily, then this diet exceeds her estimate by about 250 calories.

ANNA'S NUTRIENT INTAKE

Carbohydrate intake	300 grams	1,200 calories
Protein intake	74 grams	296 calories
Fat intake	64 grams	576 calories
ENERGY INTAKE		2,072 calories

In our weight-loss-diet-oriented society most people would look at Anna's diet and say, "You are taking in too many calories. You need to cut back, especially on the fat. Why don't you eliminate the cheese and the almonds?" This book offers another perspective: Why doesn't Anna keep her diet the same and add exercise?

If she walked for an hour (at 3.5 miles per hour, or 17 minutes per mile), she would use approximately 300 calories. At the same time she would receive all the benefits associated with exercise: increased fitness, increased quality of life, and prevention of early death. Although she may not be able to exercise for an hour when she begins, she should be able to work up to that level. As her fitness level improves, she can increase the intensity of her exercise and expend the same number of calories in a shorter period of time. For example, if she walks faster and covers a mile in 13 minutes, she would expend approximately the same amount of calories in 45 minutes as she used to in an hour.

Take-Home Message: Be physically active for at least 30 minutes every day. If you can, increase to 60 minutes every day for the most benefits.

Another reason that Anna should include exercise first rather than decrease her food intake is that she would lose nutrients if she eliminated certain foods. If Anna eliminated the cheese, she would eliminate her best source of calcium. The almonds provide her with an excellent source of vitamin E. Granted, Anna could make adjustments in her diet to substitute some lower-fat foods that still contain the needed nutrients, but the point is this: Don't automatically think about restricting food. There may be another way to keep your energy intake balanced.

At 5'6" and 130 pounds, Anna may be lulled into a false sense of security about her fitness. People tend to judge fitness based on weight and erroneously assume that a thin person is always fitter than a fatter person is. Studies have shown that this is not always true. Fatter people who are fit are healthier than thin people who are physically unfit. Anna might look at the BMI chart and assume that she is at a healthy weight as long as she is below 155 pounds (a BMI of 25 for her height). She would be wrong because her risk increases if she gains more than 10 pounds, even if her total weight is below a BMI of 25. Anna needs to begin exercising and balancing her food intake with her activity level. Recommendations for exercise are given in the following table.

EXERCISE RECOMMENDATIONS

How often?	How much?	Example
Every day	At least 30 minutes of low-intensity exercise	Moving your body, such as gardening or walking around the mall
At least 3 times per week	20 to 60 minutes of aerobic exercise	Doing an activity that increases your heart rate, such as fast walking, tennis, playing soccer, bicycling, or running
At least 3 times per week	5 to 10 minutes of stretching	Stretching before and after aerobic exercise
At least 2 times per week	15 to 30 minutes of strength (resistance) exercise	Lifting weights

Ellen is 5'5" tall and weighs 140 pounds. She walks with a friend four mornings a week before she goes to work and usually goes for a long walk on either Saturday or Sunday. They are not the fastest walkers in the neighborhood, but they are not the slowest either. Ellen works at the mall as a salesperson, which means that she stands nearly all day. Evenings usually are reserved for watching TV or lying in bed reading. She is active but does not do high-intensity activity. By using the guideline (140 pounds × 15.5 calories per pound), Ellen calculates that she needs approximately 2,170 calories per day. Her estimated daily energy intake is approximately 2,200 calories (see the following table). Her energy intake (food) and her energy output are nearly equal. If she continues this diet and activity pattern, she would expect to change her body weight very little.

ELLEN'S NUTRIENT INTAKE

Carbohydrate intake	332 grams	1,328 calories
Protein intake	69 grams	276 calories
Fat intake	66 grams	594 calories
ENERGY INTAKE		2,198 calories

At 5'5" and 140 pounds Ellen has a BMI of about 23. At this weight she falls into the healthy weight category. Given that her blood pressure, blood glucose, and blood lipid levels are within the normal range, she is at a low risk for developing several chronic diseases. She needs to continue to focus on remaining physically active and eating a healthy diet.

To meet both our nutritional and physical activity needs, a healthy diet must also contain adequate water and fluids, the subject of our next chapter.

Chapter 9

Water and Fluids

Water and fluids, including tea and (within reason) alcohol, contribute to a healthy diet. In some respects, water should be the first nutrient discussed in any nutrition book. Water makes up approximately 60% of your body's weight; you cannot live without water for more than a day or so. Mild dehydration can result in fatigue, and severe dehydration can result in death. Something so important should not be left to chance!

For many people the first time they think about water in their diet is when they start to feel thirsty. Thirst is a reflection of dehydration, not a predictor of dehydration. By the time you feel thirsty, you have already lost about 2% of your body water. If you feel thirsty, stop and drink about 16 ounces of water to reverse your present state of dehydration. Then resolve to change your drinking habits so that you don't get dehydrated and experience thirst again.

Take-Home Message: Balance water intake with water loss.

Water losses must be balanced with water intake. You obtain water by drinking liquids, consuming food, and storing water left over from chemical reactions as a result of the body's metabolic processes. But the amount created from metabolism is small—about 1 to $1^1/_2$ cups daily. Food provides about 3 to four 4 cups of water per day. Because you lose at least 6 cups a day through sweating, breathing, and urinating, you must drink liquids daily. However, the need for water is usually much greater than 6 cups a day. Environmental temperature and physical activity are two factors that can substantially change your body's need for water. **The general recommendation for adults of all ages is to drink 8 to 12 cups of fluid daily.** If you exercise in the heat, you will need more fluid to replace the amount of water lost through sweat.

You should take a scale weight before exercise and a scale weight immediately after completing exercise. Subtract the postexercise weight from the pre-exercise weight. For each pound of water weight lost (the difference in the weights is a loss of water, not a loss of fat), consume 3 cups of water. The three cups of water is in addition to the 8 to 12 cups recommended daily. Another way to determine whether you are adequately rehydrated is to check the color of your urine. It should be clear or very light yellow. Dark yellow or orange urine is a sign of dehydration.

> *Take-Home Message: Exercise in the heat requires a lot of fluid. Drink an additional 3 cups of water for each pound of weight lost in sweat.*

One confusing point is the use of the terms *water* and *fluid*. Water, mineral water, diet soft drinks, and tea or coffee without any added ingredients are fluids that are 100% water. It is reasonable to count these beverages as cups of fluid. In the past, it was recommended that caffeinated beverages such as coffee or soft drinks not be counted toward total fluid intake because the caffeine acted as a diuretic—that is, it resulted in the loss of body water. Newer studies have not found this to be true. Until more research is conducted, a reasonable approach is to consider caffeinated beverages as fluid intake. If caffeinated beverages are a large percentage of your total fluid intake, it would be wise to consume fluids at the higher end of the recommended guideline (12 cups a day for sedentary people). Soft drinks, fruit juices, and milk are about 80 to 90% water but they also contain sugars, so these beverages usually do not quench your thirst. You probably can't go wrong if you drink at least 8 cups of water every day.

Many people choose to drink bottled water rather than water from the tap or a well. You may like the taste of bottled water because it is not disinfected with chlorine as many tap waters are. Carefully reading the labels of bottled water will help you to decide which one to buy. Bubbling or sparkling waters contain carbon dioxide (either naturally or added). Mineral water contains a variety of minerals including calcium, magnesium, and sodium and has a taste that is appealing to some people, whereas distilled water has minerals removed. Spring water means that the water originally came from a spring or well.

Drinking an adequate amount of fluid is associated with good health because dehydration is prevented or delayed and the volume of urine is adequate. Low urine volume is a risk factor for kidney stones. When fluid intake is low, urine volume is low; the compounds that form kidney stones are more concentrated in the low volume of urine. Some studies have also shown a correlation between low fluid intake and an increased incidence of bladder, prostate, kidney, and testicular cancers. No risks appears to be associated with drinking 8 to 12 glasses of water a day.

Water isn't the only fluid that you can drink. Tea is a popular beverage that can contribute nutrients to a healthy diet.

Tea

Although native to Southeast Asia, tea is grown in more than 30 countries around the world. Green and black teas both originate from the same plant, *Camellia sinesis,* but are processed differently. Green tea is a result of steaming the freshly harvested tea leaves. In the production of black tea the leaves are allowed to dry until they are about half of their original weight. The dried leaves are then crushed, which stimulates a fermentation process that changes the chemical composition. Fermentation gives black tea its characteristic flavor. Nearly 80% of the tea consumed worldwide is black tea.

Both green and black teas contain polyphenols, compounds known to have antioxidant properties. Green tea contains epicatechin, a simple polyphenol. Black tea contains theaflavin and thearubigin, complex polyphenols produced through the fermentation process. Although both green and black teas contain polyphenols, the exact compositions of green and black teas are different.

Because of their antioxidant properties, polyphenols may play a role in decreasing the risk for heart disease and some cancers. Most of the studies have been conducted in Asia and have used green tea. Only a few studies have used black tea. Animal studies have shown that both green and black teas are associated with heart disease and cancer prevention. Some, but not all, human studies of green tea have shown lower heart disease and cancer rates. Similar results in humans have been found for black tea, although the number of studies of black tea is small. Animal and human studies have not found any harmful effects associated with drinking either green or black tea.

At the present time the role of green or black tea in preventing cancer or heart disease is promising, but it is too early to make specific recommendations regarding the type or amount of tea that you need to consume. Animal studies have often used high levels equivalent to a human intake of more than 10 eight-ounce cups daily. However, polyphenols are also found in red wine, grapes, apples, and oranges; so the amount of tea that you would need to consume for health benefits may be dependent on other foods in your diet. If you like green or black tea, include it in your diet.

Water and other fluids contribute to a healthy diet. Alcoholic beverages, in moderation, can also make a healthy contribution.

Alcoholic Beverages

Alcoholic beverages fall into a different category than other beverages. Although these fluids also have a high percentage of water, they are not counted toward the 8 to 12 cups of fluid recommended daily. The alcohol in beverages acts as a diuretic, and the consumption of alcohol results in increased urination. Alcohol consumption increases your chances of dehydration.

Many people wonder whether alcohol is a health hazard or a health benefit. The amount of alcohol consumed is the key issue. Alcohol is a hazard to health when it results in addiction, aggressive behavior, poor judgment (especially in automobiles), suicides, and homicides. From the perspective of health, a moderate alcohol intake is associated with a decreased risk for heart disease and death from heart disease. An intake greater than moderate is associated with an increased risk for heart disease, some cancers, and death from these and other diseases. **A moderate intake of alcohol is usually defined as one drink per day for women and one to two drinks per day for men.**

Health information about alcoholic beverages generally uses the word *drink* to describe quantity. One drink contains a half-ounce of ethanol, the form of alcohol found in alcoholic beverages. One drink is defined as 3 to 4 ounces of wine, 10 ounces of a wine cooler, 12 ounces of beer, or 1^1/$_2$ ounces of hard liquor (e.g., whiskey). **A more precise recommendation is 10 to 20 grams of ethanol daily.** A 120-milliliter (4-ounce) glass of wine contains 12.4 grams of ethanol.

So, if you drink alcohol will you live longer or die sooner? The analysis of more than 50 studies has led scientists to conclude that when people who don't drink alcohol are compared to people who consume alcohol moderately, those who consume a moderate amount live longer. The risk of premature death is sharply increased when ethanol consumption is high. The benefits of ethanol are clearly associated with moderate ethanol intake. Moderate consumption cannot be overemphasized.

Take-Home Message: Moderation in all things—especially alcohol.

Moderate ethanol intake appears to reduce the risk for heart disease (still the number one cause of death in the United States) by increasing high-density lipoprotein production. Lipoproteins are cholesterol carriers, and high-density lipoproteins tend to pick up cholesterol from the walls of the arteries and transport it to the liver, where it can be broken down. This is in contrast to low-density lipoproteins, compounds that also transport cholesterol but have a tendency to carry cholesterol to arteries of the heart and deposit it there. An increase in high-density lipoproteins lowers heart disease risk.

Higher than moderate levels of ethanol intake are associated with increased cancer risk. The risk of moderate ethanol intake on breast cancer has been controversial. Some studies have shown that one to two drinks per day increase the risk of breast cancer in women. Other studies have not found an association between one to two drinks daily and an increase in breast cancer. If you are a woman, it is probably best that you talk directly to your doctor about alcohol intake and your individual risk for breast cancer.

Red wine has received much attention as a health-promoting beverage. In addition to ethanol, red wine contains phytochemicals, notably polyphenols and phenolic acids, which are antioxidants. The antioxidant activity of 5 ounces of red wine is equal to about 2 cups of tea. Polyphenols are also found in a variety of fruits and vegetables, but red wine is a much more concentrated source. Dark grape juice and nonalcoholic red wines are alternatives for people who choose not to consume alcoholic beverages. White wine does not compare to red wine in polyphenol content because the skins of the grape are removed early in the process of making white wine.

How Am I Doing So Far?

Anna realizes that she needs to drink at least 8 cups of water daily. She drinks 1 cup of grapefruit juice and 1 cup of tea at breakfast and tends to drink iced tea at lunch, during her break, and at dinner. She feels that she drinks "a lot," so she was surprised to find that she does not consume the recommended 8 cups of water daily. Anna could improve her diet by drinking at least 2 cups of water in addition to the fluids she already consumes. If she begins to exercise, she will need to increase her fluid intake some more.

ANNA'S FLUID INTAKE

Food	Fluid
2 slices whole-grain toast	
1 poached egg	
1 cup grapefruit juice	1 cup
1 cup black tea	1 cup
1 cup split pea soup (add water to dehydrated soup)	
3½-inch bagel	
1 tablespoon peanut butter	
3-inch apple	
Iced tea (8 oz)	1 cup
Granola bar	
Iced tea (8 oz)	1 cup
2 flour tortillas	
½ cup pinto beans	
1½ oz cheddar cheese	
½ cup tomato salsa	
15 tortilla chips	
3 small carrots	
Iced tea (16 oz)	2 cups
2 scoops (slightly more than a cup) low-fat frozen yogurt	
1 oz almonds	
TOTAL SO FAR	6 cups

Ellen has gotten into the habit of drinking bottled water throughout the day. When she went to Europe she noticed that nearly everyone carried a water bottle. Once she got into the habit she found that she missed it if she didn't drink water throughout the day. An added benefit of drinking two glasses of mineral water with a high calcium content is that she would add about 100 milligrams of calcium daily to her diet. Exercise in the heat presents the greatest problem for Ellen. She often doesn't realize that she needs more water until she starts to feel thirsty.

ELLEN'S FLUID INTAKE

Food	Fluid
1 cup instant oatmeal	
1 cup nonfat milk	
1½-oz packet of raisins	
Hot water with lemon	1 cup
Baked potato with skin (approximately 7 oz)	
2 oz American cheese	

Salad bar:
    3 pieces Romaine lettuce
    8 cherry tomatoes
    2 flowerets of cauliflower
    4 red pepper strips
    1 tablespoon sunflower seeds
    1 tablespoon Italian dressing	

16 oz diet soft drink	2 cups
32 oz bottled water (throughout the day)	4 cups
8 oz orange juice	1 cup
10 Dutch Twist pretzels	
1 cup spaghetti noodles	
1 cup canned meat sauce	
2 slices French bread	
½ cup canned green beans	
1 cup mineral water	1 cup
1 cup microwave popcorn	
1 oz pistachios	
1 cup mineral water	1 cup
TOTAL SO FAR	10 cups

As you can see, planning a healthy diet by choosing nutritious foods is something that anyone can do. Once you know the nutrients that you need and the foods that contain those nutrients, it is not so difficult. An exciting aspect is that there are so many possible combinations.

Chapter 10

Putting It All Together: Carbohydrates, Proteins, Fats, Vitamins, Minerals, and Water

In a nutshell, you can eat a nutritious diet by including complex carbohydrates; whole grains; protein foods; fats from fish, nuts, and vegetable oils; lots of fruits and vegetables (especially those containing vitamin C and beta-carotene); and plenty of water. Calcium-containing foods are also an important part of every adult's diet. Being physically active allows you to take in more food and still maintain your weight. The more healthy food that you take in, the more nutrients that you will likely consume and the better your chances are that you will meet your iron and other nutrient needs.

Changing your diet is not easy, and many people find it best to start by making a few small changes. The following is an example of changes you could make that would improve your diet.

Eat more fruits and vegetables. Study after study has shown the benefits of fruits and vegetables, especially those containing vitamin C and beta-carotene. Try to include some cruciferous vegetables too.

Drink more fluid. If nothing else, improve your diet by drinking more water daily.

Be more physically active. People who exercise can consume more food without changing their weight. Generally, the more food that you eat the more nutrients that you consume.

Eat more fiber. Adding fruits and vegetables will automatically add fiber to your diet. Choosing whole-grain breads and cereals will substantially increase your fiber intake.

Experiment with beans and legumes. What's so difficult about buying a can of baked beans?

How Am I Doing So Far?

Anna and Ellen's diets are used throughout this book to illustrate the concept of building a diet. The final analysis is shown in the following table. (The complete figures are shown in appendices L and M.)

Anna's diet is adequate in carbohydrates, fiber, proteins, vitamins A and C, and calcium. Her diet is low in vitamin E and iron, although she still consumes about 90% of the amount recommended for these two nutrients. Because this is just a snapshot of her total diet (analysis of a one-day diet is useful, but a better approach is to analyze at least three days), these nutrients may not be of great concern. The more critical areas are lack of exercise, imbalance between energy intake and energy output, and lack of water intake.

Anna's diet is analyzed for additional nutrients, as shown in the following table. The pattern is the same as the previous one—most of the nutrients are adequate except for vitamin B_6 and potassium, which are low on this day. On days when she has chicken, she consumes sufficient vitamin B_6. On days when she has bananas, she consumes sufficient potassium. Also, a variety of fruits and vegetables daily, including bananas, would increase her potassium intake to recommended levels.

ANNA'S ACTUAL AND RECOMMENDED NUTRIENT INTAKES COMPARED

Nutrient	Anna's intake	Recommended intake	Compared to recommended
Carbohydrate	301 grams	300 grams	OK
Fiber	33.5 grams	At least 25 grams	OK
Whole grains	3 servings	3 servings	OK
Protein	74 grams	~50 grams	OK
Fat	64 grams	67 or less	OK
Vitamin A	2953 mcg	700 mcg	OK
Vitamin C	135 mg	75 mg	OK
Vitamin E	13.6 mg	15 mg	Low
Iron	16 mg	18 mg	Low
Calcium	1096 mg	1000 mg	OK
Water	6 cups	8-12 cups	Low
Exercise	Sedentary	20 minutes of aerobic exercise at least 3 days per week	Low
Energy intake vs. output	Energy intake higher than output	Balanced intake and output	Out of balance

ANNA'S ACTUAL AND RECOMMENDED
NUTRIENT INTAKES COMPARED (CONTINUED)

Nutrient	Anna's intake	Recommended intake	Compared to recommended
Thiamin	2.0 mg	1.1 mg	OK
Riboflavin	1.9 mg	1.1 mg	OK
Niacin	16 mg	14 mg	OK
Folate	577 mcg	400 mcg	OK
Vitamin B$_6$	1.14 mg	1.3 mg	Low
Magnesium	398 mg	320 mg	OK
Zinc	10 mg	8 mg	OK
Potassium	3118 mg	3500 mg	Low
Sodium	2696 mg	Up to 6000 mg	OK
Cholesterol	258 mg	Less than 300 mg	OK

Anna should look at her diet from two perspectives: the foods that helped her meet the recommended amounts of nutrients and the nutrients in which she fell short of the recommendations. Both are important to improving her diet and planning changes. Some foods provided a large percentage of her total daily intake for a given nutrient. For example, 1 cup of grapefruit juice provided more than 50% of her vitamin C intake. If she had consumed apple juice instead of grapefruit juice, she would have fallen short of the amount of vitamin C recommended daily. The carrots provided 85% of her vitamin A intake. Without the carrots, she would have consumed about 400 micrograms of vitamin A, much less than the recommended 700 micrograms.

Eating a variety of foods is important, so it is best not to depend on just one food to provide a particular nutrient. On the other hand, you must know which foods have about the same amount of a particular nutrient so that you can eat a variety of foods and still meet your nutrient needs. In Anna's case 1 cup of orange juice or a large serving of broccoli would provide a day's supply of vitamin C.

This analysis also points out areas that are in need of improvement. Anna is sedentary, and her energy intake exceeds her energy output. She needs to drink more water, a nutrient that will need even more attention as she begins to exercise. Four nutrients were slightly low: vitamin E, vitamin B$_6$, iron, and potassium. Including foods high in these nutrients (appendix D) would help her meet recommended levels.

Ellen's diet meets the recommended intake for all of the nutrients listed which proves that nutrient needs can be met through diet alone. It is important to note that she reached some of these recommendations by eating highly fortified foods. Without the high levels of iron and zinc in the instant oatmeal, Ellen would have fallen short (although not by much) of the recommendations for these nutrients. Also noteworthy is the convenience of Ellen's diet. She ate easy-to-prepare meals, made wise choices when purchasing lunch, and ate nutritious snacks. Her challenge will be to eat a variety of foods that provide similar nutrients and maintain her level of exercise as she gets older.

ELLEN'S ACTUAL AND RECOMMENDED NUTRIENT INTAKES COMPARED

Nutrient	Ellen's intake	Recommended intake	Compared to recommended
Carbohydrate	332 grams	300 grams	OK
Fiber	36 grams	At least 25 grams	OK
Whole grains	3 servings	3 servings	OK
Protein	69 grams	~50 grams	OK
Fat	66 grams	67 or less	OK
Vitamin A	1759 mcg	700 mcg	OK
Vitamin C	218 mg	75 mg	OK
Vitamin E	15.9 mg	15 mg	OK
Iron	24 mg	18 mg	OK
Calcium	1153 mg	1000 mg	OK
Water	10 cups	8-12 cups	OK
Exercise	Walking	20 minutes of aerobic exercise at least 3 days per week	OK
Energy intake vs. output	Intake equal to output	Balanced intake and output	OK
Thiamin	2.8 mg	1.1 mg	OK
Riboflavin	2.1 mg	1.1 mg	OK
Niacin	25.6 mg	14 mg	OK
Folate	773 mcg	400 mcg	OK
Vitamin B_6	3.3 mg	1.3 mg	OK
Magnesium	416 mg	320 mg	OK
Zinc	9 mg	8 mg	OK
Potassium	4134 mg	3500 mg	OK
Sodium	4183 mg	Up to 6000 mg	OK
Cholesterol	71 mg	Less than 300 mg	OK

Up to this point the examples have been female. Anna (age 26) and Ellen (age 45) can be compared because most of the basic nutrient requirements are the same. They can follow the same principles even though they choose different foods within each category. But what about nutrient requirements for men? Is healthful eating for men considerably different than it is for women?

Chapter 11

Healthful Eating for Men

In many respects men have an easier time meeting their nutritional needs than women do. When compared to women, men need the same amount or slightly more of all of the vitamins. The same holds true for the minerals with one exception: iron. Men need considerably less iron than premenopausal women do. The average man needs to consume more calories daily than the average woman does because men have more muscle and other lean tissue (such as bone mass). The greater caloric consumption makes getting the needed nutrients easier.

Think of calories the way you think of spending money. Money is used to buy the essentials (like food, housing, and utilities) as well as the nonessentials. Once you pay for the essentials, you can think about what nonessential items you would like to spend your money on. A person who has more spending money buys the essentials and still has money to spend on the nonessentials, some of which will be purely for pleasure. In this sense, calories can be thought of as a currency that buys nutrients. When you have more calories to spend, you can get the essentials and still have a little left over for the nonessentials (i.e., foods that don't provide as many nutrients). Both men and women must balance their caloric intake with caloric expenditure, but getting the essentials while still having some left over is more likely for men than it is for women.

A sedentary man needs about the same amount of calories as an active woman, a vivid example of the differences in caloric requirements. However, no one is suggesting that a sedentary lifestyle is healthy, even if you balance intake with expenditure and can maintain your weight. An active man needs about 2,800 calories daily. It is not difficult to meet nutrient requirements with 2,800 calories.

The basic guidelines are not based on gender. Thus, for men and women the components of a healthy diet are the same: fruits, vegetables, whole grains, beans, legumes, fish, nuts, and oils. Men need more calories and, in some cases, more nutrients than women do. Men can meet these greater needs easily by eating larger portions of healthy foods. The following example is a case in point.

Michael is a 31-year-old computer programmer. He works odd hours depending on the current project. One week he may work 8-hour days and the next week he may work 14-hour days. When under a tight deadline, he eats and sleeps in his office. He considers himself an adventuresome eater, but cooking is pretty much limited to heating leftovers in the microwave. He uses exercise as a way to break the monotony and tension of work.

Can Michael be a healthy eater? Yes, as long as he makes the right choices. In the following example, Michael eats a quick breakfast—one toaster waffle and a cup of fat-free soy milk—before going to work at 9:00 A.M. At 1:00 P.M. a coworker goes to the local deli and picks up lunch. By this point Michael is very hungry, so he orders two tuna sandwiches on whole-grain bread, a three-bean salad, and a banana. At 7:00 P.M. he realizes that he has not eaten since lunch, and someone makes a run to the local Chinese restaurant. He eats large portions of stir-fried vegetables with tofu, cashew chicken, and steamed rice. He has half a mango for dessert and hot Chinese tea. At midnight he and some of the other programmers go across the street to a 24-hour gym and play basketball for an hour. He buys a trail mix snack from the vending machine and eats it on his way home. He arrives home about 1:45 A.M.

Michael met all of his nutrient requirements by eating fruits, vegetables, whole grains, beans, fish, nuts, and oils. (The complete nutritional breakdown is in appendix N.) The choices he made were wise choices. For example, the soy milk he drank was calcium fortified. This is important because Michael does not eat dairy products and without the fortified soy milk his calcium intake would be low. He chose whole-grain bread for his sandwiches rather than white bread. He had a bean salad rather than chips with his sandwiches. The dishes he chose from the Chinese restaurant were among the most nutritious because they supplied lots of vegetables, tofu, and some nuts. The mango was an important source of vitamin A. He drank water throughout the day and exercised intensely for an hour.

Had he not chosen carefully, Michael's diet could have been lacking nutrients. If he had chosen to eat sweet and sour pork and fried rice instead of the vegetables and steamed rice, he would not have met all his nutrient requirements. If he had gone home after work instead of playing basketball, he would not have been physically active all day. But it is possible to have a healthy lifestyle even if you eat out a lot *if* you make the right choices.

The choices you make about the foods you include in your diet should reflect your understanding of the nutrients you need. The amount of nutrients that you take in should balance your energy needs. That's part of the logical approach to good nutrition. It doesn't matter whether you prepare every meal yourself or join what seems like everyone in town at the local restaurant. Making the right choices means asking the right questions.

Chapter 12

Should I Not Eat . . .?

People ask, "What should I eat?" A good starting point is fruits, vegetables, whole grains, beans and legumes, fish, nuts, vegetable oils, and water. In fact, most people don't ask what they *should* eat; they ask what they *shouldn't* eat:

Should I not eat meat?

Should I not drink milk?

Should I not eat sugar?

Not eating usually means that your nutrient intake will be lower. Before you eliminate foods from your diet, know the nutrients that you will also eliminate. The following information briefly addresses some of the most common "should I not eat" questions.

Should I not eat meat? When red meat is included in the diet it provides a source of protein, iron, and zinc. Depending on the portion size, the cut of meat, and its method of preparation, it can also provide significant amounts of cholesterol and saturated fats. Meat eaters are wise to choose small portions (4 to 9 ounces a day) of lean cuts of meat. In this case the meat serves as a source of protein, iron, and zinc; but the portion size and the cut of meat limit the amount of cholesterol and saturated fat. Some lean cuts of meat are extra-lean hamburger, flank steak, and lean pork roast.

If you don't eat meat, the important question is how can you obtain the protein, iron, and zinc that you need. Obtaining these nutrients shouldn't be a problem. Chicken and fish are good sources of protein and iron. The portion size guideline, 4 to 9 ounces daily, still applies, however. Preparation methods are also an important consideration. Fried chicken and deep-fried fish add considerable amounts of fat to your diet. Milk and milk products provide protein but are a poor source of iron. A variety of beans, legumes, nuts, and whole grains will contribute protein, iron, and zinc. The emphasis is on the word *variety*. Nonmeat eaters should be able to obtain the nutrients found in meat by eating other foods.

Take-Home Message: Lean red meat can be part of a healthy diet, but you don't have to eat meat to have a healthy diet.

Note that you don't have to have meat to have a healthy diet. Vegetarians can obtain the protein, iron, and zinc that they need; but as they restrict their animal sources of protein (meat, chicken, fish, eggs, and milk), they need to plan their diets more carefully. Vegetarians often adopt a nonmeat diet as one part of their healthy lifestyle, which includes daily physical activity, moderate alcohol intake, and abstinence from tobacco.

The bottom line is that you do not have to eat red meat to have a healthy diet but lean red meat can be part of a healthy diet. It's your choice. Remember to ask the important question, "If I don't eat red meat, what nutrients will I be missing and what foods will I need to eat to provide those nutrients?"

Should I not drink milk? You may wonder whether milk is not well suited for adults or whether milk contains hormones or antibiotics that are harmful. Perhaps you have not consumed milk for many years and you are wondering whether you will have problems if you start drinking it again. The following information should help you to address those concerns.

When milk is included in the diet it provides a source of calcium, protein, riboflavin, vitamin B_{12}, vitamin A, and vitamin D. In the United States milk is fortified with vitamins A and D. Milk may also be fortified with a few grams of additional protein. It can also provide significant amounts of saturated fats and cholesterol, depending on the fat content. Milk drinkers who choose nonfat (also called skim) milk receive the same nutrients as they would from higher-fat milks (whole milk, 2%, or 1% milk) but without the saturated fats and cholesterol.

Milk contains many nutrients, so if you don't drink milk you must find other sources of these nutrients. How easy is that? With the exception of calcium, it's pretty easy. Vitamin D can be converted from ultraviolet light, and vitamin A is found in many foods. Vitamin B_{12} is only found in foods from animal sources. If you include animal foods in your diet you will consume Vitamin B_{12}. If you do not consume any animal foods then you will need to eat a plant food that is vitamin B_{12} fortified, such as soy products. Milk is a good source of riboflavin, and people who consume milk and milk products get about half of their riboflavin from these foods. People who don't drink milk can get riboflavin from foods that have riboflavin added, such as breads and cereals. Although milk is a good source of protein, nondairy sources of protein are abundant in the United States.

Most of the nutrients in milk can be obtained easily from other food sources. The biggest problem for most people who don't drink milk is finding alternative calcium sources. Milk is such a concentrated source of calcium (about 300 milligrams in an 8-ounce glass) that when you eliminate milk or milk products, meeting your calcium requirements becomes more difficult. But it is not impossible, as shown earlier in chapter 5. The bottom line is that you don't have to consume milk to have a healthy diet, but you do need to consume enough calcium.

The reality is that most adults are lactose intolerant (that is, they can't tolerate milk or milk products because their bodies are not able to process the lactose). Ninety percent of Asians are lactose intolerant, as are 80% of Native Americans and African Americans. The majority of people from the Mediterranean countries and about half of all Hispanics are lactose intolerant. In fact, the only group of people who can consistently tolerate milk as they age are Caucasians of northern European heritage.

Lactose intolerance is a result of the body's decline with age in the production of the enzyme lactase. Lactase is needed to break down lactose, the predominant sugar in milk. About 85% of adult Caucasians of northern European heritage maintain their production of lactase. Thus, these adults can tolerate milk at almost any age. However, for the majority of adults, lactase production declines, and if they drink milk the lactose is not broken down and digested. Bacteria in the gastrointestinal tract use some of the lactose as an energy source, and this causes gas to be released. The lactose that is not used by the bacteria attracts water. For these reasons people who are lactose intolerant and drink milk often have gas, bloating, and diarrhea.

For most adults lactase production is low, not absent. Low lactase may mean that 4 ounces of milk on cereal may be tolerable, but 8 ounces of milk would be too much and would cause gastrointestinal upset. Some lactose-intolerant people can tolerate fermented milk products (such as yogurt or cheese that has been aged through bacterial action) because the lactose has been broken down during the fermentation process. They may have enough lactase to break down the remaining lactose in aged cheese or yogurt but not enough to break down the amount of lactose in milk. These people may obtain some of their calcium from fermented milk products and the remainder from non-dairy products.

Because the breakdown of lactose is a digestion problem involving lactase, people can usually tolerate milk if it has been treated with lactase. Milk that has been enzymatically treated can be purchased, although it is more expensive than nontreated milk and does not taste exactly the same. Lactase in the form of pills or drops can also be purchased and added to milk and milk products at the time they are consumed. If lactose-intolerant people want to consume milk, these products are reasonable alternatives.

You may be wondering whether people with lactose intolerance are prone to osteoporosis. Not necessarily. The key for those with lactose intolerance is consuming enough calcium. Some studies have shown that as long as calcium intake is adequate, the amount of calcium in bones is similar between those who can't absorb lactose and those who can. A chart outlining various strategies that you can use to meet your calcium requirement is found in chapter 5.

Even if you can tolerate milk and milk products, you may wonder whether you should consume them. Is there a relationship between milk intake and diseases such as arthritis and cancer in adults? Could you receive hormones or antibiotics in levels that have a negative effect on your health? At the present time the scientific literature does not show a relationship between milk intake and arthritis or cancer. The effects of hormones given to dairy cattle (bovine growth hormone [BGH] or bovine somatotropin [BST]) were debated and studied in the 1980s. One concern was the possibility of increased hormone levels in milk and, if increased, their effect on humans. A second concern was the presence of antibiotics in the milk. (As a result of BGH and BST use, antibiotic use in dairy cattle was increased because of a higher incidence of mastitis.) The scientific literature shows virtually no research in the 1990s on the safety of milk with regard to hormones or antibiotics. If these issues are a concern for you, and you decide to eliminate milk from your diet, be sure to substitute other foods that provide the nutrients that the milk formerly provided.

If you haven't consumed milk or dairy products for several years, and are not allergic to milk, the best advice is to start slowly and see if you experience any problems. Use the same principles as you would if you were introducing a new food to a toddler: Introduce only one new food at a time. Consume a small amount of the new food, but don't change other aspects of your diet. Then watch for any reactions such as stomach upset.

Should I not eat sugar? The sugar that people are referring to is the white sugar used to sweeten foods. White sugar is used to sweeten most homemade foods. Food manufacturers add white sugar as well as other sweeteners such as corn syrup and high-fructose corn syrup. There is nothing inherently bad about sugar. It is pure carbohydrate and it tastes good. But it only contributes one nutrient to your diet— carbohydrate. Sugar contains no vitamins, minerals, or fiber. Carbohydrate is not a difficult nutrient to get in your diet, so based on nutrient content alone there is no compelling reason to add sugar to your diet. However, foods with added sugar taste good, and eating good-tasting foods is part of a healthy diet.

Sugar has come under a lot of fire because as sugar consumption has increased (and it is at an all-time high in the United States), rates of obesity have increased to an all-time high. However, at the same time that sugar consumption has increased, fat intake has increased, total caloric intake has increased, and exercise has decreased. Any one of these factors or a combination of factors could result in increased body fat. Studies do not show that there is a direct correlation between sugar intake and obesity.

Take-Home Message: Keep an eye on your sugar intake—it's easy to overconsume!

Studies do show that adults up to age 55 are taking in the majority of their sugar in the form of regular soft drinks. The biggest sugar contributors for people older than 55 are cookies and cakes. The average American consumes about 328 calories per day from sugar (this figure does not include the sugars in fruits or milk). Based on average energy (caloric) intake, this is about 16% of the total energy consumed daily. Adults over 65 take in less sugar, about 12% of their total energy intake.

How much sugar should you take in? **One guideline recommends 6 to 10% of total energy.** The average adult in the United States, regardless of age, exceeds this guideline. **The Food Guide Pyramid recommends 6 to 18 teaspoons daily,** depending on your caloric level (see following chart). One teaspoon of sugar contains 4 grams of carbohydrate. A 16-ounce regular soft drink contains 52 grams of carbohydrate, the equivalent of 13 teaspoons of sugar. Per capita sugar consumption in the United States is 32 teaspoons per day.

"Should I not eat sugar?" is a simple question. The simple answer is this: Don't eat too much. If your diet is like that of most Americans, you are getting too much sugar from regular soft drinks, other sweetened drinks like fruit punch, sweetened breakfast cereals, candy, cookies, cakes, jams and jellies, honey, and sugar that you add to your food. A limited daily intake of these foods will bring your diet into line with the recommendations.

GETTING A HANDLE ON SUGAR

Recommended sugar intake for a 1,600-calorie diet	6 teaspoons daily
Recommended sugar intake for a 2,000-calorie diet	12 teaspoons daily
Recommended sugar intake for a 2,800-calorie diet	18 teaspoons daily
Per capita sugar consumption	32 teaspoons daily
Sugar content of a 16-oz regular soft drink	13 teaspoons
Sugar content of a 16-oz sport drink	4 teaspoons
Sugar content of 1 tablespoon of jam	3.5 teaspoons

We also should consider the healthfulness of packaged and prepared food. A variety of food options are available when the demands of work and busy schedules leave us short on time. Restaurants offer dine-in and carry-out foods. How do we know what we're eating when someone else has done the cooking?

Chapter 13

Restaurant Eating

Fast-food restaurants are a standard feature of the U.S. landscape. For the most part, fast-food restaurants have few items that contain fruits, vegetables, whole grains, beans, fish, nuts, and oils. The most predominant fast food meal—hamburger, fries, and a soft drink—contains a large amount of calories, sugar, and fat. Although fast-food restaurants offer some nutritious choices, such as a grilled chicken salad, most fast-food meals do not provide the nutrients needed for a healthy diet. The smell of deep-fat-fried food is particularly tempting, so even people who intend to order a salad often change their minds.

Restaurants also serve large portions. "Supersizing" has resulted in extra-large servings of fries and unlimited amounts of soft drinks. Many health professionals think that the cheap, calorie-laden food at fast-food restaurants is a major factor in the "supersizing" of the U.S. population. For healthier eating, eat at fast-food restaurants occasionally, not routinely; and order regular, not supersized, portions.

Many people find that preparing and eating meals at home is one of the best ways to consume a healthful diet. It puts you in control of portion size and makes it easier to eat a variety of healthy foods. But the reality for most people is that they frequently eat out. There are a few practical guidelines that can help people choose healthier restaurant meals.

Portion size. The norm in restaurants is large portions. Unless you are a very active person, eating the standard-size restaurant meal makes balancing food intake with exercise very difficult. Splitting a large meal with someone else is one strategy for keeping restaurant portions at a reasonable size. However, many restaurants will charge you extra for the second plate. Eating half the meal and bringing the rest home also works well.

Ethnic foods. Many restaurants serve traditional foods from countries that are known for having a healthy native diet. Asian restaurants have many vegetable dishes to choose from. Tofu and nuts are often added to dishes. Greek restaurants feature lentils, beans, and a variety of vegetables. Mexican restaurants offer vegetable fajitas and pinto beans. Unfortunately, many traditional meals are "Americanized" and have added fat. For example, traditional Mexican beans are not smothered in cheese, and deep-fried tortilla chips are an American twist. Seek out a restaurant with traditional ethnic foods, and you'll be likely to find some healthy (and tasty) items on the menu.

Ask for special preparation. Part of the fun of restaurant dining is that you don't have to prepare the food or do the dishes! Although you have given up food preparation for that meal, it doesn't mean that you can't influence it. Don't be afraid to ask for substitutions or changes. You can ask that the cook go easy on the cheese and add more veggies to your pizza. Or ask if there is a fruit or vegetable substitute for the usual side of fries. Tweaking the menu to make the meal healthier is possible, and most restaurants are happy to accommodate your requests.

Take-Home Message: Split a large restaurant meal with a companion so that the portion size is reasonable.

Restaurant dining can be a financial drain and makes it more difficult for you to follow a nutritious diet plan. With a little advanced planning, even the busiest person can prepare food at home.

Chapter 14

A Trip Down the Grocery Store Aisles

The average supermarket has thousands of products to choose from. It is no wonder that people are sometimes overwhelmed by the thought of going to the grocery store. You can get in and out of the grocery store quickly and choose foods that promote a healthy diet by doing "perimeter shopping" and focusing on a few other aisles.

Most grocery stores are set up in the same pattern. Around the perimeter of the store are fruits and vegetables, milk and milk products, meat, fish, poultry, and sometimes bread. Usually one aisle is devoted to pastas, grains, and dried beans; canned beans usually are with the canned vegetables. Cereals take up another aisle. Making a list of healthy foods that are staples in your diet will help you save both time and money at the grocery store.

So far we have covered the nutrients that you need for a healthy diet and the foods that contain those nutrients. Certain foods form the foundation of a healthy diet, and you should eat them every day. What about the other foods? Well, they are foods that you have occasionally. The next chapter helps you identify everyday and occasional foods by helping you be a savvy label reader.

Chapter 15

Everyday Foods and Occasional Foods

Fresh fruits and vegetables are everyday foods. Whole grains are everyday foods. Water is an everyday food. Beans and legumes are everyday foods. Every day you need protein, calcium, and iron; you have a lot of foods to choose from that will provide those nutrients. It is not hard to find everyday foods in the grocery store.

But what about all the other foods that are in the grocery store? If you want to have a healthy diet, many foods in the grocery store are not everyday foods; they are occasional foods. Occasionally you will want cake, cookies, and candy. Occasionally you will want chips, dip, and soft drinks. Occasionally you'll want ice cream with chocolate syrup. The key is to be able to say honestly that you only have it occasionally. If you honestly can't remember the last time you had it, then it probably is an occasional food. If you have cake on your birthday but at few other times throughout the year, then it is an occasional food. The everyday foods keep you healthy, and the occasional foods are an added treat.

An important concept to keep in mind is the influence that exercising has on your food intake. When you exercise you need more calories to maintain your weight than if you don't exercise. Physically active people often comment that exercise allows them to eat more of the occasional foods and still keep their weight in balance.

Building a healthy diet is all about making good choices. Making good choices about packaged foods requires label reading.

Be a Label Reader

If you read the labels on the packaged foods that you buy, you will learn a great deal about the nutrients they contain. The Nutrition Facts label is shown in appendix H. The following are some things to be aware of as you read the label.

Serving size. This is the amount that is in a single serving and is the basis for the nutrient information that follows. Just below the serving size is the amount of servings in the package. It is important to determine whether you are likely to consume more than one serving. If you do, adjust the nutrient information to fit the size of the portion you consume. For example, if the container serving size is $1/2$ cup but you will eat a 1-cup portion, then multiply the nutrient values by 2.

Nutrient amounts and Percent Daily Values. At the top of the label, total calories and calories from fat are listed. More important, below the dark lines amounts of nutrients are listed. All labels must list total fat, saturated fat, cholesterol, sodium, total carbohydrate, dietary fiber, sugars, and protein. Percent Daily Value (DV) also appears. The Daily Values for some nutrients appear near the bottom of the panel. Since some foods contain none of these ingredients, the percent DV may be zero.

Percent Daily Values must also appear for vitamin A, vitamin C, calcium, and iron. Percentages may also appear for other nutrients if they make a significant nutrient contribution (above 2% of the DV). Unfortunately, the grams or milligrams of these nutrients do not appear, just the percent DV. That makes the nutrient information more difficult to use because there is nothing on the label to tell you the Daily Value for those nutrients. (The Daily Values for these nutrients are listed in appendix F.)

The percent Daily Values for the vitamins and minerals do give you clues to the nutrient content, but they are best used to compare similar foods or to determine whether a food is an excellent source of a particular nutrient. For example, a food with a DV for calcium of about 30% has approximately the same amount of calcium as an 8-ounce glass of milk. A food with a DV for iron of about 13% has approximately the same amount of iron as 5 ounces of tuna.

Ingredient list. Finally, be sure to check the ingredient list, which must list ingredients in descending order by weight. Knowing that the predominant ingredients are listed first gives you information about what the product contains.

Health claims. The Food and Drug Administration approves health claims that appear on the labels. The claims help you know more about the food in general. If you know what the claims mean you will also

HOW TO DECIPHER HEALTH CLAIMS ON FOOD LABELS

Label claim	General meaning is	Specific meaning is
Calcium and osteoporosis	The food is high in calcium.	The food contains at least 200 mg of calcium.
Fruits and vegetables and cancer prevention	For fresh fruits and vegetables, the food must be low in fat and a good source of fiber. For processed fruits and vegetables, the food must be low in fat and a good source of fiber and vitamin A or vitamin C. The fiber and vitamins must be naturally occurring and not added by the manufacturer.	A fresh fruit or vegetable must contain 3 grams or less of fat and 2.5 to 4.9 grams of fiber per serving. In addition to the above nutrients, processed fruits or vegetables must contain 10 to 19% of the Daily Value for either vitamin A or vitamin C.
Dietary fat and cancer prevention	The food must be low in fat.	The food must contain 3 grams or less of fat per serving.
Fiber-containing grain products, fruits, vegetables, and cancer prevention	The food must be low in fat and a good source of fiber.	The food must contain 3 grams or less of fat and 2.5 to 4.9 grams of fiber per serving.
Saturated fat and cholesterol and coronary heart disease	The food must be low in total fat, saturated fat, and cholesterol.	The food must contain 3 grams or less of fat, 1 gram or less of saturated fat, and 20 mg or less of cholesterol per serving.
Oatmeal or oat bran and coronary heart disease	The food contains oatmeal or oat bran; is high in soluble fiber; and is low in total fat, saturated fat, and cholesterol.	The food must contain 20 grams of oatmeal or 13 grams of oat bran. In addition, it must contain 1 gram of soluble fiber (gummy fibers that dissolve in water). The food must contain 3 grams or less of fat, 1 gram or less of saturated fat, and 20 mg or less of cholesterol per serving.
Fruits, vegetables, and grain products that contain fiber, especially soluble fiber, and coronary heart disease	The food is high in soluble fiber and low in total fat, saturated fat, and cholesterol.	The food must contain .6 gram of soluble fiber (gummy fibers that dissolve in water). The food must contain 3 grams or less of fat, 1 gram or less of saturated fat, and 20 mg or less of cholesterol per serving.
Sodium and hypertension	The food is low in sodium.	The food must contain 140 mg or less of sodium per serving.
Folate and birth defects of the brain and spinal cord	The food is a good source of folate and contains a maximum of 100% of the Daily Value of vitamins A and D. (Excess amounts of vitamins A and D consumed by pregnant women can cause birth defects.)	The food must contain 10 to 19% of the Daily Value of folate while not exceeding 100% of the Daily Value for vitamins A and D.

know more about the nutrient content of the food. Some of the health claim labels and their meanings are listed in the chart on the previous page.

Learning to read labels is like learning a foreign language. The more you use it, the more comfortable you become with it. Another way to learn about a food's nutrient content is to check the manu–facturer's Web site. Many companies list complete nutrient information for their products.

Food First, Then What?

As stated in the introduction to this book, food is the vehicle by which you get the majority of your nutrients. The focus of the first part of this book is on what you should eat rather than on what you shouldn't eat. It is a positive approach to diet. Caloric intake isn't over-emphasized. Regular physical activity is a must, and balancing activity and food intake is important. You're learning how to get the nutrients you need from food.

Because your goal is to be healthy, the first step is to focus on the foods that provide the nutrients to maintain health and prevent chronic disease. But it may not be possible or practical to obtain all your nutrients from food. After you've focused on foods, the next step is to focus on supplements. Part II, "Focus on Supplements", will help you make wise decisions regarding supplements.

Chapter 16

Introduction to Supplements

So far this book has made a case for getting the nutrients you need from food. In many cases you consume fortified foods that have nutrients added. If you eat breakfast cereal or other highly fortified products (such as energy bars), you are getting the equivalent of a low-dose multivitamin and mineral supplement. But what about the hundreds of supplements available for purchase? How do you know whether you need them? How do you know which supplements to choose? How do you know how much to take?

Just as you should choose food wisely, you should choose supplements carefully. Food and supplements are not mutually exclusive. In fact, you should not consider a supplement without first determining whether you obtain that nutrient—and how much of it you obtain—from the food that you eat. The word *supplement* means "to add to," so the logical first step is to determine the amount in your diet. The amounts in supplements can be much greater than the amounts in food, so the next step is to know how much is too much and the problems associated with excess intake.

There are many reasons that it might be appropriate to take a dietary supplement. You may need a supplement to treat a nutrient deficiency. For example, if you have been diagnosed with iron-deficiency anemia, you will likely be told to take an iron supplement. This supplement will reverse your iron deficiency and build back your iron stores. If you have a milk allergy, you may be unable to add enough nondairy foods to your diet to meet your recommended calcium intake. If you are a vegetarian woman, you may be unable to obtain enough iron from nonmeat sources. You may want to take supplements to improve your overall health. You may need to consume a supplement to prevent nutrient deficiencies because you are unable or unwilling to make dietary change. Let's face it: Some people eat poorly, and important nutrients are missing in their diets.

Regardless of your reasons, if you are considering taking supplements you need to know more information about them. This book provides you with facts to make an informed decision. Two critical questions need to be answered about any dietary supplement you are considering taking: Is it safe? Is it effective? You, not any government agency, are responsible for determining both. Safety is critical—don't be lulled into a false sense of security by thinking that if a supplement is available for sale, then it must be safe. You can buy dietary supplements off the shelf that contain potentially toxic levels. Remember, just because a supplement is labeled natural (or herbal) doesn't mean it's safe or useful.

So many supplements are available that you may not know where to begin. This book breaks the vast amount of dietary supplements into smaller categories. Nutrients that are also found in food are described in chapter 19—Vitamin, Mineral, and Amino Acid Supplements. Botanical supplements, compounds that have been extracted from foods and then concentrated in pills, represent the second category. These are discussed in chapter 20. The third category covers herbs, which are extracts of plants used for medicinal purposes. Herbal supplements are presented in chapter 21.

Before 1994, the government considered herbs neither food nor drugs, but now they are considered dietary supplements. Many people use herbal supplements as alternative medications; and the number of herbal foods, which contain these alternative medications, are increasing and showing up on grocery store shelves. Chapter 21, Herbal Supplements, contains important information about herbal supplements. Specific information is given about herbal teas and herbal weight-loss products, some of which have caused harm and, in rare cases, death.

Chapter 17

Nutrients

Before deciding to add a supplement to your diet, you need to determine whether you need a dietary supplement. Let's take a few minutes to gain some perspective on the relationship between nutrients and dietary supplements. First, we'll look at how to determine the nutrients provided by your diet. We'll discuss how much you need of certain nutrients. Some people think more is better, but we'll see that this isn't always the case with nutrients. Understanding our need for nutrients will help us understand why some people need to supplement their diets.

How Much Am I Getting?

When you hear the term *dietary supplement,* think of it as "to add to the diet." First you should think carefully about your diet. How do you know whether your diet meets, lacks, or exceeds the recommended nutrient levels? Record what you have eaten for one to three days and analyze your nutrient intake. One of the best ways to do this is to consult with a registered dietitian. You can find a registered dietitian in your area by looking in the phone book, calling your local hospital, or accessing a free database maintained by the American Dietetic Association for this purpose (www.eatright.org/find.html). A dietitian can guide you through the recording process (people often make errors in recording their food intake, and a dietitian can easily spot these errors), perform a computerized diet analysis, and interpret the results of the analysis. It is money well spent.

Another way to estimate your nutrient intake is to analyze your diet yourself. Computer programs are available for purchase, and you can access several programs for free via the Internet (use the term "diet analysis" in your favorite search engine). Libraries and bookstores have books that give you this information. Once you have an estimate of your nutrient intake, you need to determine whether you are meeting your nutrient requirements through food.

How Much Do I Need?

You can determine whether you meet your nutrient requirements through food by estimating the amount you receive from food. Compare your estimated intake to the Dietary Reference Intakes (DRI) for your age and gender. The following charts list the Dietary Reference Intakes for adults. If you are not receiving 100% of the Dietary Reference Intakes, you have two alternatives. The first is to change your diet to include foods that provide the missing nutrients. The second is to consume a dietary supplement. You shouldn't do either without adequate information about the nutrients that your current diet provides.

DIETARY REFERENCE INTAKES FOR MALES

Nutrient	Males 19-50	Males 51-70	Males over 70
Vitamin A	900 mcg	900 mcg	900 mcg
Vitamin C	90 mg	90 mg	90 mg
Vitamin D	5 mcg	10 mcg	15 mcg
Vitamin E	15 mg	15 mg	15 mg
Thiamin	1.2 mg	1.2 mg	1.2 mg
Riboflavin	1.3 mg	1.3 mg	1.3 mg
Niacin	16 mg	16 mg	16 mg
Vitamin B_6	1.3 mg	1.7 mg	1.7 mg
Folate	400 mcg	400 mcg	400 mcg
Calcium	1000 mg	1200 mg	1200 mg
Iron	8 mg	8 mg	8 mg
Zinc	11 mg	11 mg	11 mg

Source: Food and Nutrition Board, Institute of Medicine, National Academies. Access at www.nap.edu.

Men of all ages need the same amount of vitamin A, vitamin C, vitamin E, thiamin, riboflavin, niacin, folate, iron, and zinc. As males age they need more vitamin D, vitamin B_6, and calcium. Males of any age who smoke need 125 milligrams of vitamin C daily, 3 milligrams more than males who don't smoke.

DIETARY REFERENCE INTAKES FOR NONPREGNANT FEMALES

Nutrient	Nonpregnant females 19-50	Females 51-70	Females over 70
Vitamin A	700 mcg	700 mcg	700 mcg
Vitamin C	75 mg	75 mg	75 mg
Vitamin D	5 mcg	10 mcg	15 mcg
Vitamin E	15 mg	15 mg	15 mg
Thiamin	1.1 mg	1.1 mg	1.1 mg
Riboflavin	1.1 mg	1.1 mg	1.1 mg
Niacin	14 mg	14 mg	14 mg
Vitamin B_6	1.3 mg	1.5 mg	1.5 mg
Folate	400 mcg	400 mcg	400 mcg
Calcium	1000 mg	1200 mg	1200 mg
Iron	18 mg	8 mg	8 mg
Zinc	8 mg	8 mg	8 mg

Source: Food and Nutrition Board, Institute of Medicine, National Academies. Access at www.nap.edu.

Nonpregnant women of all ages need the same amount of vitamin A, vitamin C, vitamin E, thiamin, riboflavin, niacin, folate, and zinc. As females age they need more vitamin D, vitamin B_6, and calcium. After menopause females need considerably less iron. Females of any age who smoke need 110 milligrams of vitamin C daily, 35 milligrams more than females who don't smoke.

Here's an example showing how a person might use the information about Dietary Reference Intakes. Jack is 55 years old. His diet analysis shows that he consumes about 800 milligrams of calcium daily from food and water. The Dietary Reference Intake for a 55-year-old male is 1,200 milligrams. Jack does not think he can change his diet to consume more calcium and has decided to take a supplement. How much of a calcium supplement does Jack need? Jack obtains the simple answer by subtracting the amount he consumes in food (800 milligrams) from the amount recommended (1,200 milligrams). In Jack's case it's 400 milligrams of calcium daily. Now that you've estimated how much of a nutrient you're consuming and compared this to what you need, you need to interpret this information.

How Much Is Too Much?

Once you know how much of a nutrient you need, the obvious question is "How much is too much?" If you obtain all your nutrients from food it would be very rare for you to get too much of any nutrient from food. If you take dietary supplements the how-much-is-too-much question is very important because you can easily take too much of a nutrient through supplementation. For any supplement that you consume you need to know the level of that supplement that can cause you harm. Scientists need to know this too, and they have the answer to the how-much-is-too-much question but only for some of the vitamins and minerals.

Tolerable Upper Intake Level (UL) has been established for 22 nutrients (listed here and in appendix P). The UL is the highest level taken daily that is not likely to cause a health problem. Intakes above the UL can be toxic. The UL assumes that you would be consuming this level daily (that is, on a routine basis).

TOLERABLE UPPER INTAKE LEVEL (UL) FOR VITAMINS ADULT MALES AND NONPREGNANT FEMALES

Nutrient	Tolerable Upper Intake Level for adult males and nonpregnant females	Based on intake from
Vitamin D	50 micrograms (mcg) daily	All food (fortified and nonfortified), water, and supplements
Vitamin A	3000 micrograms (mcg) daily	All food (fortified and nonfortified), water, and supplements
Vitamin C	2000 milligrams (mg) daily	All food (fortified and nonfortified), water, and supplements
Vitamin E	1000 milligrams (mg) daily	Fortified foods and supplements
Vitamin B$_6$	100 milligrams (mg) daily	All food (fortified and nonfortified), water, and supplements
Niacin	35 milligrams (mg) daily	Fortified foods and supplements
Folate	1000 micrograms (mcg) or 1 milligram (mg) daily	Fortified foods and supplements
Choline	3.5 grams (g) daily	All food (fortified and nonfortified), water, and supplements

Source: Food and Nutrition Board, Institute of Medicine, National Academies. Access at www.nap.edu.

TOLERABLE UPPER INTAKE LEVEL (UL) FOR MINERALS
ADULT MALES AND NONPREGNANT FEMALES

Nutrient	Tolerable Upper Intake Level for adult males and nonpregnant females	Based on intake from
Calcium	2,500 milligrams (mg) or 2.5 grams (g) daily	All food (fortified and nonfortified), water, and supplements
Phosphorus	Ages 19-70: 4 grams (g) daily Ages 70+: 3 grams (g) daily	All food (fortified and nonfortified), water, and supplements
Iron	45 milligrams (mg) daily	All food (fortified and nonfortified), water, and supplements
Zinc	40 milligrams (mg) daily	All food (fortified and nonfortified), water, and supplements
Fluoride	10 milligrams (mg) daily	All food (fortified and nonfortified), water, and supplements
Boron	20 milligrams (mg) daily	All food (fortified and nonfortified), water, and supplements
Copper	10,000 micrograms (mcg) or 10 milligrams (mg) daily	All food (fortified and nonfortified), water, and supplements
Iodine	1,100 micrograms (mcg) daily	All food (fortified and nonfortified), water, and supplements
Manganese	11 milligrams (mg) daily	All food (fortified and nonfortified), water, and supplements
Molybdenum	2,000 milligrams (mg) daily	All food (fortified and nonfortified), water, and supplements
Nickel	1 milligram (mg) daily	All food (fortified and nonfortified), water, and supplements
Vanadium	1.8 milligrams (mg) daily	All food (fortified and nonfortified), water, and supplements
Selenium	400 micrograms (mcg) daily	All food (fortified and nonfortified), water, and supplements
Magnesium	350 milligrams (mg) daily	Supplements only

Source: Food and Nutrition Board, Institute of Medicine, National Academies. Access at www.nap.edu.

Note: Use vanadium supplements with caution. There is no justification for adding vanadium to food.

Although the Tolerable Upper Intake Levels (UL) have been established for 22 nutrients, this does not mean that only these 22 nutrients have the potential to be toxic. A UL has not been established for many nutrients because insufficient scientific data are available. Always use caution when consuming dietary supplements above the Dietary Reference Intakes (DRI) unless a physician has prescribed that supplement as part of treatment. In such cases the supplement is used as a medication and the potential toxic effects are monitored. (A high amount of niacin prescribed to treat heart disease is an example of a nutrient used as medication.)

It is also important to note that the UL for many nutrients is based on your intake from all food (both fortified and nonfortified) and water as well as supplements. For these nutrients it is important to know the amount you consume from food and water as well as the amount in the supplement. A diet analysis will give you an estimate of your nutrient intake from food. You should be able to find out the mineral content of your tap water by contacting the water department where you live. (The water report will likely include the amounts of calcium and other minerals found in your local tap water. If your source of water is well water, the well water can be tested.)

Let's take another look at Jack's diet analysis. Jack has determined that he needs to consume a supplement containing 400 milligrams (mg) of calcium daily. He goes to the store and finds a reasonably priced calcium supplement; however, each capsule contains 800 milligrams of calcium. Jack needs to know if this is too much. Knowing the Tolerable Upper Intake Level (UL) for calcium can help him decide. If Jack consumes about 800 milligrams of calcium from food and water daily and takes an 800-milligram calcium supplement every day, then his total daily intake would be about 1,600 milligrams. The UL for calcium is 2,500 milligrams daily. His intake from all sources would be below the Tolerable Upper Intake Level. But Jack, like many consumers, has another question: Is more better?

Is More Better?

The Dietary Reference Intake (DRI) for calcium for a man of Jack's age is 1,200 milligrams (mg). The Tolerable Upper Intake Level (UL) for calcium is 2,500 milligrams daily. If he takes an 800-milligram calcium supplement daily, then his daily intake would be about 1,600 milligrams. That seems like a good strategy to him. Jack's logic is that 1,600 milligrams is less than the UL, so it is not too much but it is higher than the DRI; and a little bit more than the DRI is probably better. His logic is faulty and here's why. The Tolerable Upper Intake Level (UL) is not a recommended intake. It's a level at which a nutrient might harm you. The goal is not to get as close to the top without going over. The goal is to meet the Dietary Reference Intake (DRI). There is no evidence that consuming above the DRI will be of any benefit. More is not better.

Jack should look for a 400-milligram calcium supplement. It's the amount that he needs and, in this case, it has an added benefit— 400- to 500-milligram doses of calcium are better absorbed than an 800-milligram dose. Try to purchase a supplement that is closest in dose to what you need.

Another question that arises is "What might happen if I take in more than the Tolerable Upper Intake Level?" The answer depends on the nutrient.

What if I Take in More Than the Tolerable Upper Intake Level (UL)?

Exceeding the Tolerable Upper Intake Level for nutrients can have serious consequences. In some cases, such as with vitamin C, an excess dose could result in diarrhea. In other cases, such as with copper, excess doses could result in liver damage. The best advice: Don't exceed the Tolerable Upper Intake Level for any nutrient.

Are Some People Likely to Need Supplements?

Advertising of supplements is at an all-time high and is especially prevalent on television and in magazines. You may be wondering whether some people are more likely than others to need supplements. The answer is yes. Are you one of those people? The answer is maybe. Are there some people who should *not* take supplements? Yes. Are you one of those people? Maybe. Obviously, you are the only person who can answer these questions. Checking with your doctor is important, too. Who might need to take supplements? The following list identifies some groups of people who may be at risk and may benefit from supplementation.

WHO MIGHT NEED TO TAKE SUPPLEMENTS?

At-risk group	Example
People who have been diagnosed with a nutrient deficiency	Your doctor tells you that you have iron-deficiency anemia and to take an iron supplement.
People who eliminate entire food groups from their diets so that they are at high risk for a nutrient deficiency	A strict vegetarian who eliminates all animal products may need to supplement with vitamin B_{12} because B_{12} is only found in animal foods.
People who consistently take in too few calories and therefore too few nutrients	A person who frequently follows a weight-loss diet and restricts caloric intake may need a multivitamin and mineral supplement.

WHO MIGHT NEED TO TAKE SUPPLEMENTS?
(CONTINUED)

At-risk group	Example
People who take in too little of a nutrient because of an intolerance or an allergy	A person with lactose intolerance may need a calcium supplement.
Women who are pregnant	Pregnant women are encouraged to take a multivitamin and mineral supplement because the nutrient needs of pregnant women are so high.
Elderly men and women	An older person with a poor appetite, low food intake, or decreased absorption may need a multivitamin and mineral supplement.
Drug and alcohol addicts	A person who drinks alcohol instead of eating may need a multivitamin and mineral supplement.
People who take a medication that depletes the body of a nutrient	Check each medication with your physician for possible drug-nutrient interactions.

There are definitely some situations in which supplement intake could be harmful. The following chart shows a few situations where people should not take supplements.

WHO SHOULD NOT TAKE SUPPLEMENTS?

At-risk group	Example
People with liver or kidney disease	A person with liver disease experiences vitamin A and D toxicity after taking vitamin A and D supplements because the liver cannot metabolize these nutrients properly.
People who overabsorb iron	A person who absorbs too much iron may experience a toxicity if consuming iron supplements because the body stores too much iron in the liver.
People who are taking a medication that interferes with nutrient absorption, metabolism, or excretion	Check each medication with your physician for possible drug-nutrient interactions.
Smokers who consume beta-carotene supplements	In smokers beta-carotene supplements appear to increase the risk for lung cancer.

Just as there is no perfect diet, there is no perfect supplement. Even a daily multivitamin and mineral supplement may contain some nutrients that are too high given your food intake. As more highly fortified snack foods such as energy bars come on the market and you consume them, you may be taking the equivalent of a multivitamin and mineral supplement as part of your daily diet. The decision to take a dietary supplement should be based on sound principles, which are presented in the next chapter.

Chapter 18

Are Supplements Safe and Effective?

You need to gather a lot of information before you decide to consume a dietary supplement. The purpose of getting information is to be able to answer two critical questions about any dietary supplement: Is it safe? Is it effective? That's the bottom line.

We'll discuss how scientists judge the safety and effectiveness of dietary supplements. We'll learn why there is a lack of scientific information on many dietary supplements. A process is presented that will help you learn how to judge the safety and effectiveness of dietary supplements. This chapter concludes with a look at the variety of supplements covered by the dietary supplement umbrella.

The naïve consumer thinks that if a dietary supplement is for sale, then it must be safe and effective. This is simply *not true.* Dietary supplements fall under the Dietary Supplement Health and Education Act (DSHEA) of 1994. This act provides a legal definition for the term *dietary supplement,* issues guidelines for claims on the labels of dietary supplements, and specifies how product information may be used in advertising. This act does *not* ensure the safety, effectiveness, or quality of any dietary supplement!

You, the consumer, are responsible for determining whether a dietary supplement is safe and effective. You are responsible for knowing how much is too much. That is why you need as much information as you can get about any dietary supplements.

How Does a Scientist Judge the Safety and Effectiveness of a Dietary Supplement?

Scientists judge the safety and effectiveness of a supplement according to the results of scientific research. The strongest studies are those that are double-blind, placebo-controlled, performed on humans, and published in peer-reviewed journals. A double-blind study is one in which neither the study participants nor the researchers know who is receiving a treatment. Placebo-controlled means that there is a treatment group and a placebo group. A placebo is an inactive substance that resembles the treatment in every way possible. In dietary supplement research the people in the treatment group would receive a supplement and people in the placebo group would receive an inactive substance. The results of these two groups can be compared. Given that everything else is the same, any differences between the treatment group and the placebo group could be attributed to the supplement. Although animal studies produce important information, human studies are needed. Publication in a peer-reviewed journal means that the study has been scrutinized by experts (that is, reviewed by peers) who concluded that the methodology used and the authors' conclusions were sound. The peer review process helps to ensure that quality articles are published.

A single study should never be considered the definitive word. Scientists read the results of many studies and try to see how each fits into the overall picture. It is often difficult to compare studies because the study procedures differ. However, over time scientists can detect trends.

A consumer could also read the results of the scientific research. These studies are technical, and it is likely that most consumers do not have enough knowledge of the subject matter to interpret the results of the scientific studies. Consumers usually depend on health professionals to read and interpret the scientific research and report the results to consumers in a less technical style. Even with a limited scientific background consumers can learn to judge the safety and effectiveness of dietary supplements.

How Does a Consumer Judge the Safety and Effectiveness of a Dietary Supplement?

Information about supplements abounds in books, articles, and Web pages. The consumer needs to rely on unbiased sources of information. Anyone selling a supplement is not an unbiased source. This doesn't mean that the information provided is wrong, but a person who stands to benefit financially from your supplement purchase is biased. Financial gain is a powerful bias. Before you decide to take a supplement, find unbiased information. The information in this book is one source. Doctors and dietitians who do not benefit from the sale of any supplement write many unbiased articles that appear in magazines and on the Internet.

Consumers need to ask questions of health professionals about supplements. Talk to your doctor, pharmacist, or dietitian and specifically ask whether a supplement is safe and effective. You can also check some of the consumer-oriented Web sites that review dietary supplements. Look for trends. When many unbiased sources report the same recommendation, you can have more confidence in that recommendation.

The number of supplements on the shelves of grocery, drug, and health food stores is staggering. It seems that each week a different supplement is in the news. How do you know which supplements are safe and effective?

Many Dietary Supplements Lack Scientific Information

One of the problems consumers and professionals encounter is the lack of scientific information about dietary supplements. In an ideal world there would be many double-blind, placebo-controlled, human studies published in peer-reviewed journals. In the real world, supplement research is usually limited to a small number of studies. In some cases the studies have only been conducted on animals. Human studies may have a small number of subjects, so conclusions are often drawn based on the results of fewer than 100 people. An important factor to consider is the strength of the scientific research. How many studies have been published? How many people have been studied? Is there a trend that can be seen when all of the studies are considered? People on a jury are told to consider the strength of the evidence as they are deciding a defendant's guilt or innocence. Consumers must consider the strength of the scientific evidence when deciding whether a supplement is safe and effective.

When you're considering adding a supplement to your diet, a good starting point is to read the label on the supplement itself. Remember what we learned about the nutrient label on food?

How to Read a Dietary Supplement Label

You should always study the label of any supplement that you are considering taking. The Supplement Facts label (shown in appendix I) has a format similar to the Nutrition Facts label found on food.

Serving size. On the information panel are the directions for use. This is the manufacturer's recommendation for the amount that should be used and not necessarily the amount that has been shown to be effective. Similar to the information on the Nutrition Facts label, the information in the Supplements Facts box is based on the serving size listed, usually one tablet or capsule. Keep in mind that the manufacturer's directions may instruct you to take more than one tablet. If this is the case, multiply the amounts listed by the number of servings that you are taking.

Nutrient amounts and Percent Daily Values. The quantity of each supplement must be listed. Common measures are grams (g), milligrams (mg), micrograms (mcg), and International Units (IU). For botanicals and herbs, the label must indicate whether the compound is fresh or dried. If it is an extract, then the solvent used to extract the herbal ingredient must appear.

Daily Value (DV) is the amount of a nutrient needed by a person consuming a 2,000- to 2,500-calorie diet. Nutrients that have an established Daily Value, such as many vitamins and minerals, are listed first. The supplement may contain more than 100% of the Daily Value. Those compounds that do not have a Daily Value established, such as botanicals and herbs, are listed below the heavy dark line and have an asterisk (*) in the % Daily Value column. The asterisk indicates that a Daily Value has not been established.

Ingredient list. Below the Supplement Facts box is a list of the ingredients. These include both active (e.g., vitamin E) and inactive (e.g., fillers and stabilizers like gelatin and polysorbate 80) ingredients. The terms in the Supplement Facts box and the ingredient list may not match exactly. For example, vitamin E may be listed in the Supplement Facts section, but the scientific name for vitamin E, alpha-tocopherol, may appear in the ingredient list.

All the ingredients must be on the label, but they may not all appear in the ingredient list. If the ingredient appears on the display panel, it need not be listed again in the ingredient list. Read the display panel and ingredient list carefully to determine all of the ingredients in the supplement. Also, the ingredients listed on a supplement label are not required to be in order of weight or predominance as ingredients on food labels are.

Additional information. Storage instructions are given at the bottom of the panel. Supplements should be kept in a cool, dry place for maximum potency. Although it is tempting to keep dietary supplements above the refrigerator or near the stove, neither of these places is recommended. Use all of the tablets before the expiration date listed. A reminder to keep supplements out of the reach of children appears on the label. The final piece of required information is the name and address of the manufacturer or distributor.

The supplement label information is very helpful but can be confusing for consumers. For example, some supplement labels use older measures. You may read an article about vitamin D and learn that the Dietary Reference Intake is 5 mcg, but when you look at the label of vitamin D supplements you find the amount listed in International Units (IU). In the case of vitamin D, 1 mcg equals 40 IU. However, such conversions are not found on the labels. Conversions for vitamins A, D, and E are found in appendix J.

Principal Display Panel. Additional information is found on the Principal Display Panel. The brand name and number of tablets in the container must appear. The product must be identified but there are several ways that this can be done. Some products use the words *dietary supplement.* Also permitted is the substitution of the specific nutrient for the word *dietary* as well as other descriptions. *Dietary supplement, iron supplement,* or *herbal supplement with vitamins and minerals* are all allowed. If the product contains at least 100% of the Daily Value, then the words *high potency* may be used. The high-potency nutrients must be listed at the bottom of the display panel.

Health claims. Statements that describe the effect the product has on the structure or function of the body are allowed. Health claims may be made, but therapeutic claims may not be made. Consider two statements: "Calcium builds strong bones" and "Calcium restores lost bone." The first is a health claim and therefore is allowed. The second is a therapeutic claim and is not allowed. Therapeutic claims are those that involve the diagnosis, treatment, or prevention of disease. Health professionals and consumers alike often have a difficult time distinguishing between the two claims. You should be aware that the Food and Drug Administration (FDA) has not evaluated these structure or function statements. The FDA requires the following statement to appear on the label: "This product is not intended to diagnose, treat, cure, or prevent any disease."

Now that you know how to read and interpret the information on the dietary supplement label, let's look at a systematic approach to evaluating the safety and effectiveness of supplements.

Process of Evaluation

Because of the way dietary supplements are regulated (or not regulated), you, the consumer, are responsible for determining whether a dietary supplement is safe and effective. Learning how to evaluate dietary supplements is an important skill for making good decisions about your health.

A systematic approach to evaluating supplements is a multistep process. Begin by gathering information about the supplement. Organizing the information should help you to see similarities and differences in the descriptions of the supplement that you've gathered. You'll need to learn how to assess the importance of the information you've gathered; this will result in a decision about the supplement in question. Ready to get started? Let's take a look at information gathering.

Gather Information

First and foremost you must gather information to make an informed decision. Gathering information takes time and effort. Start by looking at the label of the dietary supplement you are considering taking. At a minimum, know the name of the active ingredient (or ingredients because many dietary supplements contain more than one) and the amount in each pill, tablet, or liquid serving. Check the manufacturer's recommended dose. Let's assume that you are looking at a calcium supplement. By reading the label you find that the active ingredient is calcium, the amount in each pill is 800 mg, and the recommended dose is one pill per day.

Then look for information about the active ingredient and the purpose for which you are considering taking a dietary supplement that contains that active ingredient. In this example you would want to gather as much information as you could about calcium and osteoporosis. You can get information from numerous sources including physicians, dietitians, pharmacists, other health professionals, family members, friends, magazines, newspapers, books, brochures, advertisements, and Web sites. Try to remember the source of the information.

When scientists evaluate dietary supplements, they look for trends in the data. You can look for trends in the information you've gathered.

Organize the Information

Next you need to organize the information you have gathered and look for common themes. For example, if you talked to your physician, chatted with a family member, read a magazine article, looked through a brochure, and checked several Web sites, you would find that some of the information about calcium and osteoporosis is the same regardless of the source. But you may find that some of the information is different, and you need to look more closely at the differences.

An important question to ask is "How unbiased is the source of the information?" Although much information provided by people who sell dietary supplements is correct, people who will profit from the sale of a supplement are biased. Advertisements are necessarily biased toward the product, and factual information may be overstated. The primary goal of advertisement is to highlight the advantages of a product and to increase sales of that product, not to provide unbiased educational information.

Endorsements of dietary supplements by well-known celebrities and athletes are a method used to increase sales. Endorsements are really just one person's opinion, and in many cases that person is paid to endorse the product. Friends and relatives who sell supplements may pressure you to buy them. Product endorsements, distribution bonuses, or any other economic incentives are associated with product bias and conflict of interest. It is important to get your information from unbiased sources.

After gathering and organizing the information, you may need to go back and look at the dietary supplement label again. In this example, by gathering information about calcium you would learn that calcium supplements come in different forms. Another look at the label would tell you the form of calcium found in the supplement, something you might have overlooked or not have recognized.

It's not enough to gather the information. You need to assess the relative importance of the information you have about the dietary supplement.

Weigh the Information

If you have served on a jury, you know that you will be instructed to weigh the evidence that you have heard. In court you will hear conflicting testimony and you may give more weight to the testimony of a witness who has more credibility. When you are judging the safety and effectiveness of a dietary supplement, you must also weigh the evidence. Unbiased sources of information should carry more weight than biased sources.

Because much of the information about a dietary supplement is related to how it works in the body, it is to your advantage to understand how your body works. More and more information is written for consumers about the physiological and biochemical actions of nutrients. The more you know, the better decisions you can make.

Many advertisements now include the results of scientific studies. Although many of the claims are correct, some are taken out of context or written in such a way as to be misleading. For example, an advertisement for a calcium supplement may claim, "A university study has shown that this brand of supplemental calcium helped to build strong bones." That is a correct statement, but it is taken out of context. Context is the part of a passage that surrounds the statement and determines its meaning. For the consumer, the context is the total number of calcium studies conducted. (Hundreds of studies on calcium supplements and osteoporosis have been published since 1980.) Because advertisements highlight the advantages of the product, it is common for advantageous scientific results to appear. Disadvantageous studies will not appear in advertisements. (It is unlikely that an advertisement would read, "A university study did not show that this brand of supplemental calcium helped to build strong bones.") Looking for unbiased sources that present a summary of the body of scientific literature is a consumer's best bet. (Scientific studies of calcium supplements and prevention of osteoporosis have been mixed:

Some show that supplements are helpful in preventing osteoporosis, and some show no effect on osteoporosis. Research continues; and until it has been proven that calcium supplements are ineffective, it may be prudent to take supplements because the studies have not shown any harmful effects of calcium supplementation.)

After you gather as much information as you can, you will need to evaluate the supplement you are considering taking.

Evaluate, Judge, Decide

Your evaluation of the information should help you to answer two important questions: "Is it safe?" and "Is it effective?" To answer those questions, you must consider how strong the body of scientific research is. Unfortunately, for many supplements there are only a few studies. And there may be even fewer studies that are performed on people of your gender and age who are in the same state of health and exercise to the same degree as you are.

Is it safe? Many dietary supplements sold on the market are safe; however, some are not. For supplements, as well as for medications, the dose is crucial. An often-quoted adage is "the dose makes the poison." In the case of prescription medications, you have two people who are well informed about dose: your physician and your pharmacist. When you take dietary supplements you are the person responsible for knowing whether the dose is a safe dose. Be aware that there are dietary supplements on the shelves that have doses above the Tolerable Upper Intake Levels (UL). If you are taking a dietary supplement you must know the potential safety issues and, most important, at what level the dose is "poison."

Some dietary supplements have been sold in doses that have caused medical problems and, in rare cases, death. The Food and Drug Administration reports at least 17 deaths from the dietary supplement ephedra. Millions of people have taken dietary supplements, so the number of deaths is low; but any death from dietary supplements is tragic. At least 2,000 adverse events caused by dietary supplementation have been reported to the FDA. The people who have experienced the adverse events are the ones who report the events, so the reports are difficult to interpret. But these reports do raise some cautions. If you take supplements, periodically check the Food and Drug Administration's Web site at www.cfsan.fda.gov. Under the dietary supplements heading there is a section titled "Warnings and Safety Information."

Is it effective? Once you have determined that a dietary supplement is likely to be safe, you need to know whether it works. It doesn't make sense to spend money on a dietary supplement that does not help you. In some cases many convincing studies show that a particular dietary supplement is not effective. In many cases the studies have conflicting conclusions. You may choose to take a supplement that has been shown to be promising (assuming that it has also been shown to be safe). Be sure to keep an eye out for more information as it becomes available. Wise consumers periodically re-evaluate the dietary supplements that they take.

The process of evaluation can guide you in your decision to take any dietary supplement. Once you begin to look critically at dietary supplements, you'll probably realize the magnitude of the term *dietary supplements*. The remainder of the book examines dietary supplements.

Dietary Supplement Umbrella

Throughout this book the term *dietary supplement* is used. For many years dietary supplements referred to vitamin and mineral supplements. The Dietary Supplement Health and Education Act (DSHEA) of 1994 provides a legal definition for the term *dietary supplement,* and it is much broader than the definition for vitamin and mineral supplements. A dietary supplement is a vitamin, mineral, herb, botanical, amino acid, metabolite, constituent, extract, or a combination of any of these ingredients. The term *dietary supplement* is indeed a wide umbrella.

In the next three chapters we'll take a look at many dietary supplements. Supplements of nutrients that are also found in food—vitamins, minerals, and amino acids—will be covered first. Botanical supplements will be covered next. Finally, we'll examine herbs in foods, drinks, and weight-loss products.

Chapter 19

Vitamin, Mineral, and Amino Acid Supplements

Supplemental vitamins, minerals, and amino acids are all compounds normally found in foods. This is a good place to begin our examination of dietary supplements because it is easy to compare how much you need and how much you normally obtain from food. The first group covered is the antioxidant vitamins and minerals: beta-carotene (a form of vitamin A), vitamin C, vitamin E, and selenium. Calcium and vitamin D are discussed together because they are both related to bone health. Iron receives special attention because some people should never supplement with iron. Zinc, fiber, and protein supplements are reviewed. The section concludes with information about multi-vitamin and mineral supplements.

Evaluating Beta-Carotene, Vitamin C, Vitamin E, and Selenium Supplements

Beta-carotene, vitamin C, vitamin E, and selenium are all antioxidants. In this section each will be discussed, food sources will be provided, and issues regarding safety and effectiveness will be covered.

Beta-carotene. You can get beta-carotene easily from food. Because there are so many sources, it is likely that a stop at a roadside produce stand or the supermarket produce section will result in a choice of beta-carotene foods that are flavorful and low in price. You should focus on seasonal availability. Buy apricots when they first come on the market (often one of the earliest fruits available) and cantaloupes in mid-summer. Fresh tomatoes right off the vine (gardeners always have too many and are willing to share) are a treat. Winter squashes and green leafy vegetables provide beta-carotene when fruits are not in season. Buying in season is an easy way to eat a variety of sources of beta-carotene.

Several studies have shown a connection between the intake of carotenoid-rich fruits and vegetables and lower risk for heart disease and diet-related cancers. An important point is that although beta-carotene is the best known and most studied carotenoid, it is just one of approximately 50 in foods that humans eat. Beta-carotene is an antioxidant, but it is not as powerful an antioxidant as other carotenoids such as lycopene and lutein. While scientists try to figure out just which carotenoids are needed and in what proportions, depend on fruits and vegetables to provide a variety of carotenoids.

When it became apparent that the intake of beta-carotene foods was associated with lower rates of heart disease and some cancers, scientists began studies to determine whether beta-carotene supplements had the same effect. Beta-carotene supplements were used in three large studies (between 18,000 and 29,000 subjects in each study). The studies showed that beta-carotene supplements did not reduce the risk of heart disease or cancer. In a surprising finding, beta-carotene supplements actually increased the risk of lung cancer in subjects who smoked more than one pack of cigarettes a day. The risk was so great that one study was stopped two years early. At the present time, studies do not show that beta-carotene supplements are associated with lower risk for heart disease or cancer. In the case of smokers, beta-carotene supplements appear to increase the risk for lung cancer.

You may wonder how much beta-carotene from food you should take in each day. There is no Dietary Reference Intake (DRI) for beta-carotene, only for vitamin A. When the DRI was established, there was not enough information to recommend a specific amount of beta-carotene daily. However, some researchers have suggested a daily beta-carotene intake of 6 to 10 milligrams. The typical adult intake in the United States is 0.5 to 6.5 milligrams per day, so many people fall short of the beta-carotene that they need. People who consume five servings of fruits and vegetables daily average at least 10 milligrams of beta-carotene. The following chart shows the amount of beta-carotene in some foods; however, it is easier just to remember to eat a variety of beta-carotene foods every day.

AMOUNT OF BETA-CAROTENE IN FOOD

Food	Beta-carotene (mg)
3 small apricots	6.6
1 medium spear of cooked broccoli	1.0
$^1/_4$ cantaloupe	2.2
2 medium raw carrots	7.2
1 cup cooked chard	3.4
$^1/_2$ cup cooked collard greens	4.4
1 cup cooked kale	8.0
3 leaves of Romaine lettuce	0.4
3 oz canned mango	13.1
1 sweet red pepper	1.7
$^1/_2$ cup cooked pumpkin	8.5
1 cup raw spinach	2.9
$^1/_2$ cup cooked butternut squash	4.5
1 small cooked sweet potato	10.7
1 medium raw tomato	0.5
$^1/_2$ cup cooked turnip greens	3.2

Because there is no Dietary Reference Intake (DRI) for beta-carotene, a Tolerable Upper Intake Level has not been established. You may wonder whether you can consume too much. At the present time it appears that the risk for beta-carotene toxicity from food is low. Those who take in high levels (between 15 and 50 milligrams daily) may experience a yellowish tint to the skin, which goes away when they reduce their intake of foods containing beta-carotene.

BETA-CAROTENE SUPPLEMENTS: ARE THEY NECESSARY, SAFE, AND EFFECTIVE?

Can you get enough beta-carotene from food?	Yes, easily. Sources include orange-colored fruits and vegetables such as apricots, cantaloupes, mangoes, carrots, winter squashes, and tomatoes. Green leafy vegetables are also excellent sources.
Are beta-carotene supplements necessary?	No. There are many tasty, inexpensive sources of beta-carotene.
Are beta-carotene supplements safe?	The safety of beta-carotene supplements is questionable, especially for people who smoke.
Are beta-carotene supplements effective?	No. Three large research studies have concluded that beta-carotene supplements do not help decrease the risk for heart disease or diet-related cancers.

With questions looming about both the safety and effectiveness of beta-carotene supplements, it is wise to get this nutrient from food, not supplements. Let's look at vitamin C, a supplement we know a little bit more about.

Vitamin C. Vitamin C, also named ascorbic acid, is found in fresh fruits and vegetables. Citrus fruits such as oranges and grapefruits are well-known sources; however, blackberries, cantaloupe, honeydew melon, kiwi, mango, papaya, and strawberries are all excellent fruit sources of vitamin C. Many vegetables also provide vitamin C. These include bok choy, broccoli, brussels sprouts, red and green cabbage, kale, kohlrabi, peppers, rutabaga, snow peas, tomatoes, turnips, and turnip greens. Some sources are particularly rich. For example, an 8-ounce glass of orange juice provides 100% of the Dietary Reference Intake for adults for vitamin C. If you choose a variety of fruits and vegetables in your diet, you should have no trouble getting the amount of vitamin C recommended.

Vitamin C may be added to foods, notably to juice drinks and juice cocktails. Cranberry juice cocktail is nearly equivalent to orange juice in vitamin C content because of the addition of vitamin C to the cranberry juice (sugar is added too). Apple and grape juices are usually fortified with vitamin C. The addition of supplemental vitamin C makes the drinks more commercially competitive with juices that have a naturally occurring source of vitamin C. The vitamin C itself is the same chemical compound whether found naturally, added by the food processor, or taken in the form of a tablet. Vitamin C in supplements is absorbed to the same degree as vitamin C in food.

Vitamin C appears to play a role in preventing heart disease, cancer, and possibly cataracts. It is a powerful antioxidant, but the functions of vitamin C in the body are varied, and its role in preventing disease may be more than just its antioxidant properties. The current Dietary Reference Intake (75 to 90 milligrams daily for nonsmoking adults) is higher than that recommended in the past (60 milligrams daily) because studies have shown a link between vitamin C and disease prevention. However, there is no compelling evidence that levels of vitamin C need to be very high (i.e., 1,000 milligrams or more) to prevent heart disease or cancer. It is also not known whether the reason for the disease prevention is the presence of vitamin C or the presence of vitamin C working with other compounds, notably phytochemicals. If it is solely vitamin C, then people should see a benefit when they obtain vitamin C from any source (food, fortified food, or supplements). If other compounds play key roles in the effectiveness of vitamin C, then there is a strong argument for obtaining the vitamin C from foods in which it occurs naturally.

In a country where adults pop vitamin C pills as if they were candy, it is important to know that the Tolerable Upper Intake Level is 2,000 milligrams daily. Consumption above this level may result in diarrhea and other gastrointestinal problems.

Vitamin C is being studied to determine its role in the prevention of heart disease, cancer, and cataracts; but you may know about vitamin C because of its link to the common cold. Current research suggests that vitamin C does not prevent colds. However, studies have shown that vitamin C may help to reduce the duration of a cold. If you take vitamin C once you have a cold (recommendations range from 250 milligrams up to 1,000 milligrams daily), remember that you are using vitamin C as an over-the-counter drug. Report your use of vitamin C supplements to your physician, and watch for side effects as you would with any over-the-counter medication.

VITAMIN C SUPPLEMENTS: ARE THEY NECESSARY, SAFE, AND EFFECTIVE?

Can you get enough vitamin C from food?	Yes, by choosing a variety of vitamin C-containing fruits and vegetables. Some foods, such as orange juice, will provide the amount needed daily in a single serving.
Are vitamin C supplements necessary?	Not for most people. However, at least 25% of adults in the United States consume less than 60 mg of vitamin C from food daily.
Are vitamin C supplements safe?	Vitamin C supplements appear to be safe if less than 2,000 mg is taken daily.
Are vitamin C supplements effective?	It is not known whether vitamin C supplements are effective in preventing heart disease, cancer, and cataracts because vitamin C may work in conjunction with other nutrients or phytochemicals. Supplements appear to be effective for reducing the severity of a cold but are not effective in preventing colds.

We know more about vitamin C supplements for reducing the severity of colds than we know about supplemental vitamin C and the reduction of chronic disease risk. Vitamin C from food is still your best bet, but vitamin C supplements are probably safe for most adults. Vitamin C supplements are popular, as are vitamin E supplements.

Vitamin E. Vitamin E is a fat-soluble vitamin that is a powerful antioxidant. The best dietary sources are vegetable oils, particularly safflower oil. Wheat germ is a concentrated source of vitamin E, and nuts and seeds have a substantial amount. Fruits and vegetables also contribute, but none is a concentrated source. Animal fats do not contain vitamin E. Fat-soluble vitamins need fat present for adequate absorption, so it is not surprising that vitamin E is found in foods that contain vegetable fats.

Estimating dietary intake of vitamin E is difficult because nutrition databases are not always accurate. Various oils are added to processed foods and listed on the label as "vegetable oils," but the vitamin E content will vary significantly based on the specific type of oil added. It is also difficult to determine how much oil is added to food as it is prepared and how much of the preparation oil is then consumed. Given all of these potential problems, the best estimate is that adult men consume approximately 9 milligrams daily and adult women consume approximately 7 milligrams daily, high enough to prevent a vitamin E deficiency but far short of the recommended daily intake of 15 milligrams.

A low dietary intake of vitamin E may be a result of a reduced-fat diet. Low-fat diets that eliminate salad dressings eliminate an excellent source of vitamin E. Nuts and seeds are also excellent sources that may be perceived as too high in fat to be included routinely in the diet.

Of particular interest is the role that vitamin E plays in reducing the risk for heart disease. There is strong support in animal studies, but studies in humans have been less convincing. Of the four largest studies in humans, one showed that vitamin E did prevent heart attacks but the other three studies did not. Most of the studies are done in high-risk populations such as smokers or those with a history of heart disease, so it is not possible to predict whether vitamin E protects against heart attack in healthy people with low risk for heart disease. For this reason many health professionals think it is too early to recommend vitamin E supplements for people who do not have heart disease. However, vitamin E supplements are popular, especially among older adults. Many people who supplement do so with 200 to 400 milligrams of vitamin E daily, and these levels are not thought to be harmful. The

Tolerable Upper Intake Level (UL) is 1,000 mg; amounts above this may increase the tendency to hemorrhage (bleed).

VITAMIN E SUPPLEMENTS:
ARE THEY NECESSARY, SAFE, AND EFFECTIVE?

Can you get enough vitamin E from food?	Yes, but it may be difficult, especially if vegetable fats are restricted.
Are vitamin E supplements necessary?	Until more accurate databases are developed and more clinical trials are conducted, it is not known whether vitamin E supplements are necessary.
Are vitamin E supplements safe?	Yes, vitamin E supplements appear to be safe if less than 1,000 mg is taken daily.
Are vitamin E supplements effective?	There is some evidence that vitamin E supplements are effective in reducing the risk for heart attacks in adults. However, the majority of studies have not found vitamin E supplements to be effective.

Two U.S. dietary habits have people wondering whether our vitamin E intake is adequate. The first habit is a low-fat diet, which consequently restricts the amount of this fat-soluble vitamin. The second is the low intake of whole grains, nuts, seeds, and other sources of vitamin E. More studies and better measurements are being released, so this is definitely a vitamin to keep an eye on. Vitamin E supplements are probably pretty safe for most adults.

Much has been written about the antioxidant properties of beta-carotene, vitamin C, and vitamin E; however, the mineral selenium is also a powerful antioxidant.

Selenium. Selenium is found in high concentrations in grains, vegetables, and fish. Meat and dairy products also contain selenium, but absorption is lower than with other sources. The Dietary Reference Intake (DRI) for adult males is 70 micrograms (mcg) daily. Adult non-pregnant females need 55 micrograms (mcg) per day. Intake in the United States appears to be adequate.

Several studies have shown that adequate selenium is associated with decreased risk for some cancers, notably prostate cancer. The amount of selenium in these studies ranged from 40 micrograms (mcg) daily (easily obtainable from food) to 200 micrograms (mcg) daily (obtained through supplements). It is not clear whether selenium works by itself or in conjunction with other nutrients such as vitamin E.

Selenium is known to be toxic at high levels. The Tolerable Upper Intake Level (UL) has been established at 400 micrograms (mcg) daily. This figure includes all food, water, and supplements; but drinking water does not contain significant amounts. Selenium toxicity results in selenosis, a condition in which nails and hair become brittle and fall out.

SELENIUM SUPPLEMENTS:
ARE THEY NECESSARY, SAFE, AND EFFECTIVE?

Can you get enough selenium from food?	Yes. Grains, vegetables, fish, meat, and dairy products are sources. The soil in the United States is not selenium deficient.
Are selenium supplements necessary?	No, sufficient selenium can be obtained from food.
Are selenium supplements safe?	Selenium supplements up to 300 micrograms appear to be safe.
Are selenium supplements effective?	It is not known whether selenium supplements are effective in preventing cancer because selenium may work in conjunction with other nutrients or phytochemicals that are present in food.

Although lesser known than the other antioxidants, selenium is an important nutrient that helps the body to offset the problems that result from oxidation. If you supplement, remember that selenium is known to be toxic at high levels and it is important not to exceed the UL.

Now let's look at a widely used mineral supplement, calcium, and a vitamin that helps in calcium's absorption, vitamin D.

Evaluating Calcium and Vitamin D Supplements

Try to obtain calcium from food first. Milk and milk products such as cheese and yogurt are the best food sources of calcium. Green leafy vegetables such as broccoli, kale, and turnip greens also provide calcium; but the amount of calcium per serving is substantially less than with a serving of milk. Soy products, such as calcium-fortified soymilk and tofu preserved with calcium sulfate, often contain added calcium. Other calcium-fortified products include orange juice and high-calcium milk. A variety of foods can add a small amount of calcium. On average, adults in the United States consume between 400 and 700 milligrams (mg) daily. The recommended intake is 1,000 to 1,500 milligrams daily depending on age, gender, and estrogen status. Many Americans have diets that are deficient in calcium.

Some people cannot drink milk because they have a milk allergy, or cannot drink very much milk because of lactose intolerance, or don't want to drink milk because they dislike the taste. It is more difficult but not impossible to consume enough calcium from food when milk and milk products are excluded. Calcium-fortified foods provide a calcium supplement using food as the vehicle. Calcium supplements may also be taken separately. The absorption of calcium from supplements is as good as the absorption of calcium from milk.

Supplemental calcium comes in many forms, including calcium carbonate and calcium citrate. Calcium carbonate contains the most calcium per tablet, but absorption may be lower than it is from other forms. Calcium citrate is prescribed when stomach acid is low, as is often the case with older women. Any calcium supplement is better absorbed when taken with food and when taken in 400- to 500-milligram doses. Vitamin D also increases calcium absorption.

The Tolerable Upper Intake Level (UL) for calcium is 2,500 milligrams per day; intakes above this level may result in kidney stones in people who are prone to them and high blood calcium levels resulting in kidney problems. Calcium supplements can bind with tetracycline, reducing the absorption of both substances. When bone meal, oyster shells, or dolomite (limestone) are the source of calcium, the supplement may contain contaminants such as lead.

The focus on adequate calcium intake is a result of the number of hip and wrist fractures reported in older adults. Bones contain 99% of all the calcium in your body. The remaining 1% is found primarily in your blood. Hormones strictly regulate blood calcium levels and ensure a steady supply of calcium from the blood to the muscles and nerves. If dietary calcium is not sufficient, calcium is removed from your bones to maintain blood calcium levels. Over time this removal of calcium results in osteoporosis, a condition of porous bones. Porous bones eventually shatter. Hip and wrist fractures are common in people with osteoporosis.

During childhood, adolescence, and early adulthood (up to about age 25) calcium is readily deposited in your bones. Adequate calcium at this time helps to maximize the amount of calcium stored in your bones. After age 40, calcium is slowly lost from your bones. After women go through menopause, usually around age 50, calcium loss accelerates because of reduced estrogen. Adequate calcium intake for women older than 40 may help to slow the loss of calcium from their bones and delay the onset of osteoporosis. Osteoporosis is highly influenced by genetics, which accounts for approximately 45 to 60% of the density of your bones. Calcium is a major nutritional factor, but hormones and exercise are also significant factors as shown in the following chart.

SOME RISK FACTORS ASSOCIATED WITH OSTEOPOROSIS

Nutritional	Inadequate calcium intake Inadequate vitamin D intake Excessive alcohol intake
Non-nutritional	Increasing age Gender (female) Estrogen deficiency Inadequate exercise or physical activity Smoking

Calcium supplements appear to be safe, but the effectiveness of sufficient calcium in preventing and slowing osteoporosis is still being studied. Some studies have shown that calcium and vitamin D supplements can reduce calcium loss from bones and decrease the risk for fractures in adults, including the institutionalized elderly. Other studies have not shown a protective effect. Some bone sites may be more responsive than others to supplementation. For example, within five years of the onset of menopause women who took calcium supplements slowed the loss of calcium from the radius (the outer bone of the arm) but not the spine. While research continues and until supplementation is proven to be ineffective, it is wise for those with low dietary calcium intake and several risk factors for the development of osteoporosis to use calcium supplements.

Calcium absorption and metabolism requires the presence of vitamin D. Unfortunately, vitamin D activity declines with age, and the lack of vitamin D affects the amount of calcium absorbed and retained in your body. Vitamin D helps transport calcium across the small intestine. Older people have less vitamin D, so calcium supplements often have vitamin D added to make sure that calcium absorption can take place. Vitamin D also influences calcium retention. When blood calcium levels are low, vitamin D signals the kidney to retain the calcium that would otherwise be lost in your urine. Because calcium and vitamin D work hand in hand, the two are often found in the same supplement.

Vitamin D is available in food and can also be converted by the body from ultraviolet light (sunshine). Milk is fortified with vitamin D and is an excellent source. Exposure to sunshine for 15 minutes to 3 hours daily (dark-skinned people need greater exposure than light-skinned people) also provides sufficient vitamin D. Direct exposure is necessary because ultraviolet light cannot penetrate window glass or heavy clothing. If you are always indoors or you are completely covered with heavy clothing and sunscreen when you are outdoors, you may develop a vitamin D deficiency over time. As you age your body's ability to convert ultraviolet light to vitamin D declines.

In the absence of sufficient sunshine exposure, your body depends on vitamin D from food sources. Adults need between 5 and 15 micrograms (mcg) from food daily. Vitamin D is one of the most toxic vitamins, so you should not exceed the Tolerable Upper Intake Level of 50 mcg daily. Serious damage to the heart and kidneys can result from continued excessive levels. Vitamin D used to be measured in international units (IU). If you see this measurement, remember that 2,000 IU is equal to 50 micrograms (mcg) of vitamin D. Vitamin D is a logical addition to a calcium supplement because it helps increase calcium absorption.

CALCIUM SUPPLEMENTS: ARE THEY NECESSARY, SAFE, AND EFFECTIVE?

Can you get enough calcium from food?	Yes, if you consume enough milk and milk products. Possibly, if you consume a variety of high-calcium foods in place of milk and milk products, but it is more difficult No, if milk and milk products and other high-calcium foods are excluded.
Are calcium supplements necessary?	Those who do not obtain sufficient calcium from food may need calcium supplements.
Are calcium supplements safe?	Supplemental calcium, in the form of calcium-fortified foods and calcium tablets, appears to be safe as long as total calcium intake (food and supplements) is below 2,500 mg daily.
Are calcium supplements effective?	Possibly. Study results vary.

A QUICK TEST FOR CALCIUM SUPPLEMENTS

Calcium supplements should dissolve fast enough so that the calcium will be available for absorption as it passes through the gastrointestinal tract. A simple test is to put the calcium supplement in 4 ounces of vinegar. Stir occasionally. After 30 minutes the pill or tablet should be dissolved.

VITAMIN D SUPPLEMENTS:
ARE THEY NECESSARY, SAFE, AND EFFECTIVE?

Can you get enough vitamin D from food?	Yes, if you consume enough milk and milk products. You can also convert enough vitamin D from 15 minutes to 3 hours of daily ultraviolet (UV) light exposure.
Are vitamin D supplements necessary?	Yes, in some cases including lack of any ultraviolet light exposure and the decline of the body's ability to convert UV light to vitamin D (common in older adults).
Are vitamin D supplements safe?	Vitamin D is one of the most toxic vitamins but it appears to be safe if total vitamin D intake (food and supplements) is not greater than 50 mcg daily.
Are vitamin D supplements effective?	Vitamin D supplements are effective in increasing the absorption of calcium in older adults.

Calcium is a nutrient that people may not get enough of, and this is especially true as people age. Aging also has an effect on people's need for vitamin D, so calcium and vitamin D supplements may be just what the doctor ordered. Be sure to stay below the UL for these nutrients, especially vitamin D, which is highly toxic at high levels.

Another common supplement is iron. But some people should never take iron, so check with your doctor before supplementing with iron.

Evaluating Iron Supplements

The recommended intake of iron is 8 milligrams daily for men and women who have been through menopause. In the United States people generally consume 5 to 6 milligrams of iron for every 1,000 calories. Thus, if you consume 1,350 to 1,600 calories daily, you probably will consume at least 8 milligrams of iron. However, nonpregnant women of childbearing age need 18 milligrams daily, and obtaining this amount of dietary iron is difficult. Dietary sources of iron are outlined in chapter 6. Because the iron demands in pregnancy are so high (27 milligrams daily), women who are pregnant are routinely prescribed a multivitamin and mineral supplement containing sufficient iron.

Iron is unique among nutrients because an easy, inexpensive blood test for hemoglobin is a direct measure of iron status. The hemoglobin test is an excellent measure of iron because 80 to 90% of all the iron that is absorbed is used to make hemoglobin. Low hemoglobin is a reflection of iron deficiency. For nonpregnant females a hemoglobin value between 11.5 and 15 g/dL (grams per deciliter) is considered normal.

The normal range for males is 14 to 18 g/dL. Values below these ranges indicate iron-deficiency anemia.

Iron-deficiency anemia is associated with feelings of fatigue and tiredness that do not improve with getting more sleep. The cause is a lack of iron, not a lack of sleep. Once diagnosed by a physician, it is easily treated with iron supplements, usually 30 to 60 milligrams daily. The iron supplements reverse the iron-deficiency anemia and replenish iron stores. Replenishment is slow, and people may need to take iron supplements for six months. Iron status is monitored when supplements are withdrawn to make sure that hemoglobin stays in the normal range.

Most males consume adequate iron in their diets and rarely develop iron-deficiency anemia. In contrast, iron-deficiency anemia is common in females of childbearing age because iron is lost from the body each month as a result of menstruation. Women who consume fewer than 1,500 calories per day are at risk for low iron intake. Women who are lacto-ovo vegetarians (i.e., avoid animal sources of iron such as meat, fish, and poultry but do consume milk and eggs) also tend to be at greater risk. Animal flesh contains heme iron, a type of iron that is particularly well absorbed.

Iron supplements should be taken between meals, not with a meal. The reason for this is that an iron supplement containing more than 25 milligrams (which is usually the case) could interfere with the absorption of zinc in the food. The iron in fortified food is less than 25 milligrams and does not interfere with zinc absorption.

The relationship between low dietary iron intake and iron-deficiency anemia is a classic example of taking in too little of a nutrient and developing a nutrient deficiency. Iron-deficiency anemia is common in females, and fatigue is always a symptom. Iron supplements are available for purchase without a prescription. So, you think that if you are feeling a little fatigued, it might be a good idea to try an iron supplement. That is a bad decision because iron supplements might be very dangerous for you to take.

About 1 million people in the United States should never take iron supplements. These people have hemochromatosis, a disease that is also known as iron overload. Most, but not all, are Caucasian males. They have a genetic predisposition to absorb too much iron. Once the iron is absorbed, the body cannot excrete it very well and the excess iron is stored in the liver and other organs and can cause many medical problems. In many cases this condition is undiagnosed so a person may not know that iron supplements would be dangerous. For your safety, do not self-prescribe iron supplements.

Think of an iron supplement as a medication that helps to treat the disease iron-deficiency anemia. As with any medication, keep iron supplements out of the reach of children. It may surprise you to know that the most common cause of fatal accidental poisoning in children under the age of three is the consumption of iron supplements. Young children are naturally curious and put many things into their mouths. Unfortunately, for many children, swallowing iron supplements intended for adults is fatal.

The Tolerable Upper Intake Level (UL) for iron is 45 milligrams daily and includes all food (fortified and nonfortified), water, and supplements. Iron supplements for the treatment of iron-deficiency anemia are generally prescribed in the range of 30 to 60 milligrams and are an example of a nutrient used as a medication. Adverse gastrointestinal distress (nausea and constipation are common) are the side effects associated with intakes above the UL. Report adverse effects to your physician.

IRON SUPPLEMENTS:
ARE THEY NECESSARY, SAFE, AND EFFECTIVE?

Can you get enough iron from food?	Yes, but it may be difficult for women of childbearing age.
Are iron supplements necessary?	Yes, by those diagnosed with iron-deficiency anemia.
Are iron supplements safe?	Iron supplements appear to be safe for most adults except for those with hemochromatosis and other iron overload conditions. Consult with your physician before taking iron supplements. Caution: Every year children die from iron overdose because they swallow iron supplements intended for adults.
Are iron supplements effective?	Yes, iron supplements taken for 4 to 6 months will reverse iron-deficiency anemia.

Iron is an example of a supplement that could be helpful or harmful depending on the person. It's unique because a blood test for hemoglobin is a good measure of iron's status, and many studies show its effectiveness in treating iron-deficiency anemia. Another mineral, zinc, is not so easily categorized.

Evaluating Zinc Supplements

Zinc is a mineral that regulates numerous processes in the body because it is part of more than 100 enzymes (compounds that speed up reactions in the cells). It has far-reaching effects, including an antioxidant function, on the cells of the body. Zinc also plays an important role in the immune system; many throat lozenges contain zinc.

The recommended daily dietary intake of zinc is 8 milligrams for women and 11 milligrams for men. The median intake in the United States is 9 milligrams for women and 13 milligrams for men. A diet that includes animal foods and sufficient energy (calories) typically supplies 10 to 15 milligrams of zinc daily. Studies have shown that impaired immune function can occur with a mild zinc deficiency.

Including more zinc-rich foods, such as red meat, milk, and seafood, is one way to increase zinc intake. Take zinc supplements with caution because they may interfere with the absorption of other nutrients, especially copper and iron. If you consume supplemental zinc, limited the dosage to 15 milligrams per day.

At least 11 studies have been conducted on the use of zinc lozenges to reduce the duration and severity of colds. Six studies showed that cold symptoms were reduced in severity or duration, whereas five studies showed no effect. Zinc lozenges contain 14 to 16 milligrams of zinc and should be used only as a short-term treatment (3 to 7 days) because zinc blocks the absorption of copper, causing copper deficiencies.

The Tolerable Upper Intake Level (UL) for zinc is 40 milligrams per day. Some zinc lozenges contain 16 milligrams each, and the instructions on the package indicate that you could take one lozenge 3 times per day. In this case you would receive zinc above the UL from just the lozenges alone.

ZINC SUPPLEMENTS:
ARE THEY NECESSARY, SAFE, AND EFFECTIVE?

Can you get enough zinc from food?	Yes, but some people consume marginal or moderately low amounts.
Are zinc supplements necessary?	Possibly by those whose diets are routinely low in zinc.
Are zinc supplements safe?	Zinc supplements of 15 milligrams (mg) or less appear to be safe.
Are zinc supplements effective?	The effectiveness of zinc supplements is unknown because study results are mixed.

So far we've covered vitamins and minerals in both food and supplements. Now let's look at another nutrient, fiber, which is also available in food and supplement forms.

Evaluating Fiber Supplements

Plenty of dietary sources of fiber exist. Whole-grain breads and cereals, legumes, fruits, and vegetables are all excellent fiber sources, and it is possible to consume the recommended amount (25 grams of fiber daily) from food sources alone. In addition to fiber, these foods contain many other nutrients. Try to obtain sufficient fiber from food first. However, in the United States the average fiber intake is less than 15 grams per day. You may have problems chewing or swallowing high-fiber foods, and a fiber supplement may help. There is no Tolerable Upper Intake Level (UL) for fiber, but if you consume more than 40 grams of fiber per day you may block the absorption of other nutrients such as calcium, iron, and zinc.

Fiber supplements usually include one of three fiber sources: psyllium, methylcellulose, or polycarbophil. Psyllium is derived from the husks of the psyllium plant and is a concentrated source of fiber. Methylcellulose and polycarbophil are made from the cell wall of plants (cellulose). They are chemically altered to make them resistant to breakdown in the gastrointestinal tract. Some supplements do not contain any of these sources but extract fiber from fruits, vegetables, and grains. At maximum dosages the supplements provide approximately 6 to 9 grams of fiber daily.

FIBER SUPPLEMENTS:
ARE THEY NECESSARY, SAFE, AND EFFECTIVE?

Can you get enough fiber from food?	Yes. Whole-grain breads and cereals, legumes, fruits, and vegetables all contain fiber (as well as other nutrients).
Are fiber supplements necessary?	Those who do not obtain sufficient fiber from food may need fiber supplements to avoid constipation. This is especially true for older adults who have trouble chewing and swallowing foods that contain fiber.
Are fiber supplements safe?	Fiber supplements are safe if used as directed. An excess amount of fiber can cause gastrointestinal problems.
Are fiber supplements effective?	Yes. Fiber supplements have been shown to be effective in reducing constipation.

High-fiber foods, plenty of fluids, and daily physical activity are all factors that will help you avoid constipation. However, many adults, especially older adults, benefit from fiber supplements.

Evaluating Protein Supplements

Protein supplements usually consist of whey, casein, and soy proteins. The same proteins from supplements are in milk, meat, fish, poultry, soybeans, and other foods that contain protein. The average adult in the United States takes in more protein than is recommended.

Protein supplements are popular with athletes who are trying to increase the size and strength of their muscles. Increasing muscle size and strength requires dedication to resistance training (weightlifting) and moderate protein intake in the presence of adequate calories. Strength athletes need about twice the amount of protein recommended for nonathletes (approximately 1.6 grams of protein per kilogram of body weight compared to 0.8 grams of protein per kilogram of body weight).

Proteins contain amino acids; amino acids stimulate muscle protein synthesis in the presence of resistance training. These amino acids are found in both protein-containing foods and in protein supplements. Most studies of resistance-trained athletes have not found that protein supplements are associated with an increase in muscle growth, and there are no studies that suggest that protein supplements are better than proteins found in food. Protein supplements may be a convenient way for athletes to consume protein, but protein foods can provide the same benefit.

Protein supplements may contribute to dehydration, low carbohydrate intake, and an increased excretion of urinary calcium. Additional water is needed to metabolize the high protein levels, thus the link to dehydration. When protein intake is high, carbohydrate intake tends to be lower. After several days of exercise a high-protein, low-carbohydrate diet will result in lower muscle glycogen (carbohydrate) stores. High protein intake also creates excess acid when the protein is metabolized. To neutralize the acid the body pulls calcium carbonate from the bones. The carbonate neutralizes the acid and the calcium is excreted in the urine, possibly contributing to osteoporosis. Those who use protein supplements are advised to drink plenty of water (check that urine color is clear or light yellow) and consume enough carbohydrate foods. Protein supplements appear to be safe for healthy adults.

PROTEIN SUPPLEMENTS:
ARE THEY NECESSARY, SAFE, AND EFFECTIVE?

Can you get enough protein from food?	Yes. Meat, fish, poultry, eggs, milk, soybeans and other vegetable proteins are abundant in the United States.
Are protein supplements necessary?	No. Sufficient protein can be obtained from food. Even athletes, who need more protein than nonathletes, can meet their protein needs through food alone.
Are protein supplements safe?	Protein supplements are probably safe for healthy adults.
Are protein supplements effective?	Most studies have found that protein supplements are not effective in increasing muscle growth in resistance-trained athletes.

Protein foods are widely available in the United States, so most people obtain enough protein from their diets. Athletes are the most frequent users of protein supplements. The body utilizes the proteins in foods and supplements in the same way, but drinking a protein supplement may be more convenient for athletes than eating protein-containing foods.

Evaluating Multivitamin and Mineral Supplements

Our food supply and our use of dietary supplements are changing. In times past, a multivitamin and mineral supplement was recommended for overcoming nutrient deficiencies that were a result of a poor diet. But more foods have nutrients added, and many people are taking supplements in addition to highly fortified foods. Scientists are considering a new dimension: the role that multivitamin and mineral supplements play in preventing disease. These changes mean that we need to rethink our use of the typical "one-a-day" multivitamin and mineral supplement.

Preventing vitamin and mineral deficiencies. For many people taking a tablet containing 100% of the recommended amount of vitamins and minerals daily relieves them of the need to eat nutritiously. Or does it? Keep in mind that there is no single solution for dietary shortcomings, not even a multivitamin and mineral supplement. The intake of a daily multivitamin and mineral supplement is probably safe and provides insurance against classic nutrient-deficiency diseases. But classic nutrient deficiencies are not a major health problem for most adults in the United States. People in this country no longer have beriberi (thiamin deficiency) or pellagra (niacin deficiency). One reason is that fortified food provides the equivalent of a multivitamin and mineral supplement. The following chart compares the amount of vitamins and minerals found in one serving of fortified cereal and one multivitamin and mineral tablet. Individual cereal and supplement brands vary. Fortified cereals usually contain at least 10 vitamins and minerals. If iron is added, then calcium may not be added; but this is not true for all cereals. Multivitamin and mineral supplements may contain 30 nutrients but not all of them at 100% of the Daily Value.

FORTFIED CEREAL AND MULTIVITAMIN AND MINERAL SUPPLEMENT COMPARED

Nutrient	Daily Value	Fortified cereal (% Daily Value)	Multivitamin and mineral supplement (% Daily Value)
Vitamin B$_1$	1.5 mg	100	100
Vitamin B$_2$	1.7 mg	100	100
Niacin	20 mg	100	100
Vitamin B$_6$	2 mg	100	100
Folate	400 mcg	100	100
Vitamin B$_{12}$	6 mcg	100	100
Vitamin C	60 mg	100	100
Vitamin A	900 mcg RE	15	100
Vitamin D	400 IU or 10 mcg	10	100
Vitamin E	20 alpha-TE or 30 IU	100	100
Calcium	1000 mg	0	16
Iron	18 mg	100	100
Zinc	15 mg	100	100

Food fortification is widely accepted in the United States and is instrumental in preventing nutrient deficiency diseases, but some scientists are raising questions about U.S. food fortification policy. The number of fortified foods is increasing. Over the years the addition of iron and zinc has increased substantially. Between 1970 and 1987 the total amount of iron added to food in the United States increased almost 20 times, and the amount of zinc added increased 32 times. Some scientists are warning about the overconsumption of nutrients because of an increase in the amount of nutrients added to food and the number of fortified foods now available in the United States. It is something to think about.

Many dietitians and physicians think that most people should be able to obtain the necessary nutrients if they eat a nutritious diet. As a general rule, if you are meeting the Dietary Reference Intakes (DRI), you should be getting enough nutrients. However, it should be noted that the DRI are based on population studies, and for a small group of people the DRI are too low to meet their individual nutrient needs. For less than 5% of the population, the DRI are not high enough because these people need much more of a particular nutrient than most people do. Unfortunately, it is extremely difficult to determine who falls into this category. Through trial and error these people discover that they need more of certain nutrients, and vitamin and mineral supplements may help. But even people with high daily nutrient needs should not consume above the Tolerable Upper Intake Level for any nutrient.

Although obvious vitamin deficiencies are rare in the United States, subclinical vitamin and mineral deficiencies are not. A subclinical deficiency is a marginal deficiency, not quite adequate and not enough for the body to have outright deficiency symptoms. It is not known how many adults have subclinical vitamin deficiencies but some, and perhaps many, do. Some laboratories can test blood for vitamin levels, but such tests are expensive and not always locally available.

Preventing chronic disease. People with subclinical vitamin and mineral deficiencies are at risk for chronic diseases such as heart disease, some cancers, and osteoporosis. The scientific studies clearly show that the intake of nutrients from foods can help prevent chronic disease, and there is some evidence that vitamin and mineral supplements can too. But the evidence that nutrients by themselves can help prevent chronic disease is not as compelling as the case for obtaining nutrients from food.

Perhaps the biggest concern is the lack of folate, vitamin B_{12}, and vitamin B_6, and the risk for heart disease. People with subclinical deficiencies of these vitamins are at greater risk for developing high levels of homocysteine in the blood. Homocysteine is an amino acid; when blood levels of homocysteine are high, the risk for heart disease is increased. Folate, vitamin B_{12}, and (to a lesser degree) vitamin B_6 are necessary for metabolizing homocysteine correctly. When these vitamins are not present, homocysteine can accumulate in the blood. Most studies have shown that supplementing these three vitamins helps lowers homocysteine in those with elevated levels.

In June 2002, authors of an article published in the *Journal of the American Medical Association* recommended that all adults take one multivitamin supplement daily as a prudent measure to prevent some of the chronic diseases. Caution was expressed about consuming excess amounts of vitamins A and D (which can be toxic) and the inclusion of iron in most one-a-day type supplements. Remember that some people should never supplement with iron. Always check with your doctor about the supplements that you are taking.

MULTIVITAMIN AND MINERAL SUPPLEMENTS: ARE THEY NECESSARY, SAFE, AND EFFECTIVE?

Can you get enough vitamins and minerals from food?	Yes, but many people do not get enough for a variety of reasons, including poor food choices.
Are multivitamin and mineral supplements necessary?	No, if vitamin- and mineral-rich foods are eaten. Yes, if energy (calorie) intake is low, if nutrient needs are exceptionally high (less than 5% of the population), or if diet is obviously deficient in nutrients.
Are multivitamin and mineral supplements safe?	Multivitamin and mineral supplements are probably safe for most healthy people, but be sure to check with your doctor.
Are multivitamin and mineral supplements effective?	Multivitamin and mineral supplements are effective for preventing nutrient deficiencies in people who have low nutrient intake. It is not yet known how effective such supplements are in preventing chronic disease.

One of the concerns health professionals have about people's consumption of vitamin and mineral supplements is that they don't realize the potential for danger. High levels of some nutrients are actually used in the medical profession as medications. This is one reason that you should always consult with your doctor about the amount of any dietary supplement that you are thinking about taking

Nutrients As Drugs

When nutrients are taken at levels greater than could ever be obtained in food, they no longer act as nutrients; they act as drugs. For example, niacin may be prescribed for disorders of lipid (fat) metabolism such as high blood cholesterol levels (hypercholesterolemia). The niacin dose prescribed is 500 to 2,000 milligrams (mg) and is substantially greater than the recommended adult dietary intake of 14 to 16 milligrams. The prescribed niacin dose clearly exceeds the Tolerable Upper Intake Level for niacin, which is 35 mg, and physicians monitor for potential toxic effects. Over-the-counter niacin products are available, but studies have shown that they are less effective than prescribed forms and have a greater incidence of liver toxicity. Talk with your doctor if you are considering taking any dietary supplement that exceeds the Tolerable Upper Intake Levels for any nutrient.

Vitamin, mineral, fiber, and amino acid supplements all have one thing in common: They are normally found in food. That means that you can evaluate your food intake and determine whether you receive an adequate amount through diet alone. It also gives you an idea about how much of a supplement you might need. But the dietary supplement market is not limited to nutrients that are found in foods. There is a large market for supplements of compounds that have been extracted from food. In the next chapter we'll take a look at some of the botanical supplements that are available for purchase.

Chapter 20

Botanical Supplements

Botanicals are compounds that have been extracted from foods and then concentrated in pills. Sometimes botanicals are distinguished from herbal supplements, but most of the time consumers use the two terms interchangeably. When the terms are used separately the term *botanical* usually refers to the compounds that are extracted by the manufacturer. When the manufacturer concentrates or otherwise processes the botanical (in other words, the raw material), it then becomes part of an herbal supplement. For the consumer, the distinction is not important.

The manufacturing process affects the safety and effectiveness of botanical supplements. In the first part of this chapter we'll explore processing practices. Then, we'll take a look at three popular botanical supplements: garlic, soy, and phytochemicals. These supplements are popular because research studies have shown that when people eat a diet containing substantial garlic, soy, or fruits and vegetables (good sources of phytochemicals), their risk for some diseases is low. An important point is that the original idea for concentrating many of these compounds came from studies of people's diets. For example, in Mediterranean countries where lots of garlic is used, heart disease tends to be lower than in United States. In Japan, a country where soy is an everyday food, breast cancer rates are low. Studies in many countries have shown that people who eat a lot of fruits and vegetables daily have a lower prevalence of some diseases.

When studies show differences in eating patterns and disease risk, it is natural to explore further. The first question that must be asked is whether the food has a substantial effect on its own or whether it is part of a larger dietary pattern. For example, is the low rate of breast cancer in Japanese women due to their soy intake alone or is it just a part of a healthy diet and lifestyle that also includes fish, lots of vegetables, and daily exercise? It is difficult to separate all the factors, but a substantial element of the diet deserves more study.

Once an individual element is identified as possibly conferring health benefits, that element (such as garlic) is researched further. Scientists and consumers want to know the how and why. What chemicals are in the garlic? How do they work? Do they only work under certain conditions? Can the chemicals be extracted and concentrated? One thing leads to another, and pretty soon the garlic used to season foods is now a concentrated garlic tablet. But the intriguing questions don't go away. Do botanicals give you the same health benefits as the food from which they were extracted? Do botanicals give you greater health benefits because they are more concentrated? Do botanicals not give a benefit because something is missing that was originally found in the food? Answers to these questions help you decide whether you should take a botanical supplement. Let's start by looking at the process by which botanical supplements are manufactured.

Good Manufacturing Practices and Dietary Supplements

The amount of active ingredient (in other words, the dose) in prescription drugs and over-the-counter medications is closely regulated, and companies that produce these medications must follow guidelines known as Good Manufacturing Practices (GMP). However, the FDA does not require dietary supplement manufacturers to use GMP. This raises concerns about the amount of active ingredient that is found in a dietary supplement, especially botanical and herbal supplements. Many studies have shown that the amount of active ingredient in dietary supplements can vary tremendously, and some cases studies have shown that there is no active ingredient in the botanical or herbal supplement tested.

An important issue for any medication or dietary supplement is that the active ingredient has been standardized. This means that the amount found in the supplement is the same as the amount found in a laboratory standard. Let's say that the standard for a supplement is 1% active ingredient. That means that every supplement produced in every batch should contain 1% active ingredient. Dietary supplement manufacturers who voluntarily use Good Manufacturing Practices would have a system that ensures that every dietary supplement sold is standardized. However, in the absence of required GMP there are dietary supplements on the market whose active ingredient is above or below the standard or not present at all.

Standardization is important, especially in botanicals and herbs, because so many factors can affect the amount of active ingredient present. The amount of active ingredient depends on the part of the plant used (the leaf has a different amount than the stem), the species of the plant, the age at harvest, the way the plant is prepared (cutting gives different results than mashing), the processing (dried or not dried), and the methods used for extraction. No wonder the amount of active ingredient could vary so much! Without standardization there is little chance of producing a consistent dose of active ingredient.

Systems are now being put in place by which supplement manufacturers who follow Good Manufacturing Practices can receive a certification. Certification is a tool that consumers can use to make sure that they are purchasing supplements that reflect GMP. Look for certifications by organizations such as the NNFA (Trulabel program), USP (USP seal), NSF International, ConsumerLab, or other organizations that provide independent verification of dietary supplement GMP. (NNFA is the National Nutritional Foods Association, USP is the United States Pharmacopeia, NSF International is the National Sanitation Formulary International, and ConsumerLab is ConsumerLab.com.)

Now that you have some understanding of the importance of standardization of the active ingredient in a botanical supplement, let's take a look at three types of botanicals, beginning with garlic.

Evaluating Garlic Supplements

Garlic has been used for thousands of years to season food. Garlic bulbs contain alliin, a biologically inactive and odorless compound. Crushing, thinly slicing, or chewing garlic allows alliin to come in contact with an enzyme (allinase) that converts alliin to allicin. Allicin is a biologically active compound that has a characteristic odor.

Studies to date suggest that the consumption of raw or cooked garlic protect against stomach and colon cancer. This protection is probably a result of the antibacterial activity of garlic in the stomach as well as the presence of anticancer compounds found in the garlic cloves. Studies show that garlic supplements do not appear to protect against these cancers, but the number of studies is small.

In addition to protecting against stomach and colon cancer, garlic has been shown to have a limited effect on lowering cholesterol in the first one to three months of use. It may also decrease platelet aggregation, which helps to keep blood clots from forming. But the studies have raised more questions than they have answered. Chief among them is whether a garlic supplement is the same as fresh garlic. At the present time there is more scientific evidence for the use of fresh garlic than there is for garlic supplements.

How much garlic needs to be consumed to be beneficial to health? In the United States no recommendation has been made. German Commission E, a panel of experts who review herbal formulations in Europe, suggests that approximately one to two cloves daily (approximately 4 grams by weight) may be beneficial, but this level is really a guess because the scientific literature is so scant. The commission requires that garlic supplements sold in Europe contain the equivalent of 2,700 milligrams (2.7 grams) of fresh garlic. Garlic supplements do not appear to be harmful.

The use of fresh garlic daily is unappealing to some people because they do not like the taste or the odor associated with garlic. This odor stays on the breath and can be dissipated through the skin. Consumer demand has motivated supplement manufacturers to pursue odorless garlic supplements.

Remember Jack? If Jack goes into the grocery store to look at garlic supplements, what will he find? Probably a lot of different brands to choose from. In this example, 11 supplements were on the shelf as shown in the following chart. These are the supplements that were on the shelf of a large grocery market store when a random search was made. The information was copied from each label, but brand name information does not appear in the chart. The purpose of the chart is to show the amount of information the consumer must deal with and not to make recommendations about the purchase or nonpurchase of a particular brand. No wonder consumers are confused when it comes to choosing a dietary supplement! Where should Jack begin?

GARLIC SUPPLEMENTS COMPARED

Serving size	Recommended dose	Ingredient	Amount	Miscellaneous information
1 caplet	1 per day	Garlic (Allium sativum) as garlic powder	520 mg = 1300 mg fresh garlic	Odor controlled
2 tablets	2 tablets up to 2 times per day	Garlic concentrate (clove)	480 mg standardized to yield 1% allicin (4.8 mg)	60 mg vitamin C 194 mg calcium 200 mcg chromium
2 tablets	1 tablet 3 times daily	Garlic powder	200 mg	
2 tablets	Up to 2 tablets 3 times per day	Garlic powder	300 mg standardized to yield 1% allicin	
1 tablet	1 daily	Garlic powder (clove)	400 mg = not less than 5000 mcg of allicin	76 mg calcium 3 mg iron
1 softgel	4 softgel tablets daily	Garlic oil (concentrated)	1 mg	Parsley seed oil (2 mg)
1 softgel	1 softgel 1 to 2 times daily	Garlic oil	3 mg	
2 tablets	Up to 2 tablets 3 times per day	Garlic clove	300 mg standardized to yield 0.8% allicin	
1 tablet	2 tablets daily	Concentrated garlic bulb	500 mg = 1,250 mg of garlic bulbs	
1 tablet	1 tablet daily	Garlic clove	400 mg standardized to yield 1% allicin	
1 caplet	1 or more as desired	Aged garlic extract powder	600 mg	

One of the best places to begin is to look at the ingredients. In this case the ingredient (garlic) is found in different forms: concentrated cloves, powder, or oil. One piece of information that could help Jack distinguish between the supplements is the form of the supplement.

Many garlic supplements contain garlic powder, which is obtained from fresh garlic cloves that are crushed, dried, and ground into a powder. Much of the alliin (and therefore the allicin) is lost in the dehydration process. Allicin is not a very stable compound; so unless the preparation is standardized to contain a designated level, there may not be any allicin in the supplement. Garlic powder in supplements is usually standardized to contain between 0.8% and 1% allicin.

Garlic oil is extracted from fresh garlic cloves. This process appears to eliminate any allicin that was present in the original cloves. It is questionable whether there is any amount of active ingredient in garlic oil that could confer a health benefit.

Aged garlic extract (AGE) is a different process than those described previously. Soaking garlic cloves in an alcohol solution produces AGE, and the extract is aged for up to 20 months. The compounds in the extract are converted to stable compounds, which are thought to be safe. An advantage of AGE is that this process has been well studied and many reports appear in the scientific literature.

If Jack decides to consider only supplements that have been standardized or contain aged garlic extract, then he has narrowed the field to five. Another point for Jack to consider is the amount of the active ingredient (the dose). In the case of garlic supplements, the amount of garlic that would be equivalent to 4 grams of fresh garlic is 9 milligrams of allicin. For some supplements the amount of allicin is noted on the label (4.8 milligrams). However, most labels do not show the amount, but the consumer can calculate it (480 milligrams × .01 = 4.8 milligrams). It may be necessary to consume more than one tablet daily to obtain the amount of allicin present in 4 grams of fresh garlic. In the case of aged garlic extract, most research studies have used 1,000 milligrams (1 gram) or more.

Jack realizes that he will need to take one tablet at least a couple of times a day if he hopes to benefit from the garlic supplement. This is not very appealing to him because he isn't much of a "pill person." Another point he considered was whether the supplement had other ingredients added. In his case, he wanted only a garlic supplement. To make an informed decision Jack had to invest some time to find out the necessary information about the active ingredient. In the end he decided not to supplement because he knew he would not be diligent about taking the supplement more than once a day, and that if he didn't, then he wouldn't get enough of the active ingredient to have an effect.

Sometimes it is tempting to close your eyes and just choose one of the supplements on the shelf; but if you do you, may not be buying a supplement that supplies a significant amount in the right form to have a beneficial effect. Remember that you are responsible for knowing whether the dose you consume is likely to be effective. It is not illegal to sell a supplement with a dose that has been shown in research studies to be too low to be effective.

Garlic is one of the top 10 most-purchased supplements. Another top 10 supplement contains active ingredients derived from soy. Soy supplements are heavily advertised to menopausal women.

Evaluating Isoflavone (Soy) Supplements

The use of soybeans in the diet has been long recognized as a way to obtain dietary protein. More recently, the use of soy proteins has been recommended as a way to reduce heart disease. Other studies have suggested that soy, because it is a concentrated source of isoflavones, may reduce the risk of breast cancer and osteoporosis. Soy has also been suggested to have a beneficial effect on the symptoms associated with menopause, specifically the reduction of hot flashes. Isoflavone supplements are available for purchase and are popular with women. Advertisements for isoflavone supplements often mention menopause, reduction in hot flashes, protection against osteoporosis, and reduction in breast cancer risk.

Soy protein receives special attention because it is such as concentrated source of isoflavones, specifically daidzein and genistein. As a rule of thumb, each gram of soy protein contains 2 to 4 milligrams of isoflavones. Soy milk and tofu contain about 2 milligrams per gram of protein. Textured soy protein contains approximately 5 milligrams per gram of protein. You can estimate the amount of isoflavones you obtain from soy, but an exact figure is not possible because of the variety of ways that soybeans are processed. If you consume 10 grams of soy protein per day, it is estimated that you would also consume 20 to 40 milligrams of isoflavones. Isoflavone supplements also vary in the range of 25 to 50 milligrams of isoflavones per tablet, and a frequently recommended dose is two tablets per day.

Daidzein and genistein, the specific isoflavones found in soy, have a chemical structure similar to estrogen. Sometimes the word *phytoestrogen* is used when referring to the compounds in soy because the isoflavones are phytochemicals and they have an estrogen-like effect. In premenopausal women estrogen helps protect against heart disease and loss of calcium from bones. An important question, then, is what role an estrogen-like compound plays.

Studies have shown that the consumption of at least 25 grams per day of soy protein decreases total cholesterol, low-density lipoprotein (LDL) cholesterol, and triglycerides in women. The reduction was modest (approximately 9% decrease in cholesterol, 13% decrease in LDL cholesterol, and 10.5% decrease in triglycerides) but is thought to contribute to a decreased risk for heart disease, the number one killer of postmenopausal women. The lipid-lowering benefit in the studies was a result of soy protein intake and not a result of isoflavone supplements. Although the isoflavones in soy protein (daidzein and genistein) are known to reduce LDL cholesterol, it is not known whether the reduction in heart disease risk is due just to the isoflavones or whether these compounds play a role in conjunction with fiber or other components of the soy. In most of the studies the soy protein replaced animal proteins, which may be another protective factor. Soy protein may be a viable alternative for those who need a modest reduction in blood lipids, so it is something to ask your physician about.

At the present time research is under way to examine the effect of soy protein and isoflavones on bone health. However, there is little evidence at this time that the consumption of soy can protect against osteoporosis or reduce the risk of fractures. Although much has been written about the ability of soy to reduce hot flashes, the scientific evidence is scant. At the present time there is not enough scientific evidence to show that soy or isoflavone supplements are effective in reducing hot flashes in all women.

Much has also been written about soy and breast cancer. Japanese women living in Japan have some of the lowest breast cancer rates in the world. These same women also consume more soy protein (the average intake of isoflavones is 30 to 40 milligrams per day) than women in Western countries. An obvious question is whether an increased intake in soy protein and therefore isoflavones could reduce breast cancer risk. At the present time the scientific literature does not support the hypothesis that the consumption of soy by adults reduces breast cancer risk.

There has also been much concern over a related issue: the possibility that soy consumption could promote tumor growth in women who have been diagnosed with breast cancer. Some studies have shown that genistein and daidzein, at low concentrations, stimulate breast cancer growth. Adding to the confusion, some studies have shown that genistein inhibits cancer growth at high concentrations. Unfortunately, the high and low concentrations are from studies of individual cells, not from studies of humans. It has not yet been determined what level of soy protein or isoflavone intake is considered high (or low) in humans. Scientists argue about whether breast cancer patients should consume soy (in hopes that high concentrations will be protective) or not consume soy (for fear that low concentrations will stimulate tumor growth). Because the studies are conflicting and more studies are being published all the time, women would be wise to seriously study the issue and talk to their physicians about their soy intake.

In some respects soy and isoflavones have become women's issues, but more attention is being paid to the role soy may play in protecting against prostate cancer. Similar to breast cancer rates, prostrate cancer rates in Japanese males living in Japan are much lower when compared to men in the United States, particularly African Americans. At present the data are limited and more research is needed.

The strongest evidence to date regarding soy is for the replacement of animal proteins in the diet with soy proteins to modestly improve blood lipids. But more studies are being conducted, and recommendations may change in the future.

Another area of active research is phytochemicals. Most days you can pick up a newspaper and read the results of a phytochemical study.

Evaluating Supplements Containing Phytochemicals

As more and more phytochemicals are being isolated from food, chances are that you will see more phytochemical supplements come on the market. Phytochemicals can be extracted from food, but the important question is "Does a phytochemical work in the same way if it is separated from the food in which it is originally found?" The answer to this question is unknown for most of the phytochemicals currently on the market, which is a strong argument for obtaining your phytochemicals from foods.

In some cases a natural source of the food is sold with additional phytochemicals. For example, green tea is a source of catechin; but some green teas have added catechins, so the tea is now a more concentrated source than in the past. The assumption is that "more is better," but this assumption is based on intuition, not on scientific studies. More may be better or it may be worse.

One of the limitations of studies of phytochemicals is that, in most cases, the particular food is studied in isolation, not within the context of the total diet. For example, red wine is a concentrated source of phytochemicals and thought to have a beneficial effect on some chronic diseases. Would the effect be the same in a person who consumed phytochemicals from many sources? Or, as one research article asked, "Is wine beneficial only in a bad diet?" At the present time the most prudent advice regarding phytochemicals is to obtain them from as many food sources as possible.

Research on botanicals will likely produce interesting information for a long time. The body of scientific literature about botanicals is changing. But one thing has not changed: the important questions to ask. Is it safe? Is it effective? Asking those questions will never go out of style. They're the same questions to ask of herbal supplements.

Chapter 21

Herbal Supplements

Although herbs have been used for thousands of years, their availability and popularity in the United States are much greater now than in the past. There are herbal supplements, herbal foods, and herbal weight-loss products. Many advertisements imply that herbal products are safer than nonherbal products. That is a claim that you should pay close attention to.

Before 1994, herbs were considered neither food nor drugs. Since the passage of the Dietary Supplement Health and Education Act, herbs are considered dietary supplements. Many people use herbal supplements as alternative medications. The key questions for all supplements (Are they safe? Are they effective?) still need to be answered, but consumers using herbal supplements as alternative medications must also ask whether the herbal supplement is as safe, less safe, or more safe than a medication taken for the same purpose.

By law, a drug is defined as an article intended for use in the diagnosis, cure, mitigation, treatment, or prevention of disease. Dietary supplements must carry the following warning on the label: "This product is not intended to diagnose, treat, cure, or prevent any disease." Drugs and dietary supplements are meant to be different. You need to ask yourself why you would take a particular dietary (herbal) supplement. For example, ask yourself, "Why am I considering taking echinacea?" If your answer is "To keep from getting a cold or the flu," then you will take it to prevent disease. Why are you taking bearberry leaves (uva ursi)? If the answer is "To get over my urinary tract infection," then you are using it to treat or cure a disease. If you are using an herbal (dietary) supplement to treat, cure, or prevent a disease, you would be wise to apply the same standards that you would use to evaluate an over-the-counter medication or a prescription drug.

Drugs and dietary supplements differ in at least two very important ways: determination of safety and effectiveness, and standardization of dose. The approval of a prescription or over-the-counter drug by the FDA requires that manufacturers conduct tests and demonstrate the drug's safety and effectiveness. The FDA continually monitors approved drugs. In contrast, dietary supplements do not require preapproval by the FDA. The manufacturer does not have to provide the FDA with any safety information as long as the ingredients were on the U.S. market before 1994. The manufacturers are not required to inform the FDA of any safety reports that surface after the product is on the market. Consumers and health professionals can report adverse events to the FDA at their MedWatch Web site at www.fda.gov/medwatch/report/hcp.htm or by phone at 1-800-FDA-1088. If you are taking a dietary supplement, check the FDA Web site to see whether any safety issues have been reported.

Lack of standardization is one of the major complaints about herbal supplements. By law a 325-milligram dose of aspirin must contain 325 milligrams of aspirin. But herbal supplements are not regulated in the same way as drugs. Just as we've seen with botanicals, the species, the part of the plant used, and the maturity when harvested influence the potency of the herbal materials used to make herbal supplements. The processing and the extraction of the active ingredients in the herb may not be standardized, so two batches made from the same raw material may have different strengths. It would be similar to buying two bottles of the same aspirin, but one would contain 325 milligrams and one would contain 125 milligrams of aspirin. Studies of some herbal supplements, including St. John's wort and ginseng, have shown that amounts varied considerably from those listed on the label. In some cases the supplements contained no active ingredients at all, and in a few cases the supplements were contaminated. There is no government agency that tests or regulates the strength of dietary supplements. Therefore, consumers must determine that the amount stated on the label is really the amount that is in the herbal supplement. It is virtually impossible for consumers to test the supplements they consume, but there are several consumer-oriented Internet sites that report results of independent testing of herbal products.

Some of the best-selling dietary supplements in the United States are echinacea, St. John's wort, ginkgo biloba, garlic, saw palmetto, ginseng, goldenseal, aloe, Siberian ginseng, kava kava, and valerian. Although these supplements are classified as dietary supplements, they are not nutrients and, with the exception of garlic, have not been traditionally consumed as foods. Because this book focuses on food and dietary supplements that affect nutritional status, these best-selling supplements (with the exception of garlic) are not covered. If you are considering taking these supplements, evaluate them as you would if you were taking a medication. Be sure to answer the three very important questions listed here:

Are they safe?

Are they effective?

Are they as safe (or safer) and as effective (or more effective) than medications taken for the same purpose?

Doctors and pharmacists are good resources in your quest for information about how herbal supplements compare to prescription and over-the-counter medications. Unfortunately, many consumers do not mention their herbal supplement intake to these professionals.

Herbal Foods

More herbal foods are coming on the market and are found on grocery store shelves. At the present time the food seems to be a vehicle for the delivery of herbal medications. The foods that contain echinacea, ginseng, ginkgo, kava, and saw palmetto do not appear to enhance the action of these compounds. One question to ask yourself is how herbal foods differ from herbal medications. The key questions are, as stated previously, as follows: Are they safe? Are they effective? Are they better than the food or medicine taken separately? Studies do not exist, so consumers must make their own judgments based on information that is known about the active ingredients in each herb.

Many herbal teas are sold for medicinal purposes. Diet teas (also known as slimming teas) have long been popular as part of weight-loss diets. Herbal teas for relieving tension or inducing sleep are plentiful. The following information will help you to evaluate herbal teas that fall into these general categories.

Evaluating Medicinal Teas

A variety of teas are available on the grocery store shelves. Black tea and green tea *(Camellia sinesis)* are brewed and consumed as a beverage in the same way that coffee is brewed and consumed as a beverage. Herbal teas, made from a variety of herbs, blossoms, spices, and other plant materials, have long been an alternative to black and green tea. You may drink herbal tea because you prefer its taste. Or you may drink herbal tea to avoid the caffeine or tannins found in green and black tea. In some cases, you may consume herbal tea because of its medicinal properties. The focus of this section is those teas that are sold for medicinal purposes.

Diet Teas

Diet teas (the word *diet* in this context refers to weight loss), also known as slimming teas, have been on the market for a long time and many have renewed consumer interest because they contain a blend of herbs. Many diet teas advertise that they no longer contain caffeine (a compound that has a diuretic effect) and imply that the added herbs are a more natural approach. But diet teas contain herbs that are known to have a diuretic effect. Herbs found in diet teas often include birch leaf, goldenrod, juniper berry, and licorice root, although many combinations are found because nearly 200 herbs are known to have a diuretic effect. The herbs stimulate urine production; the loss of urine (mostly water but also waste products) results in a small loss of scale weight. A loss of weight through loss of water is deceptively attractive to someone focused solely on a number on the scale—attractive because scale weight is lower but deceptive because no loss of body fat has occurred and the risk for dehydration is increased.

Herbal Teas for Stress Relief or Sleep

Herbal teas sold to provide stress relief or help with sleep usually contain a variety of herbs that have a calming effect on the body or are antispasmodics. Common herbs in such teas are valerian, rosemary, peppermint leaf, lavender, chamomile, orange blossoms, hops flowers, and lemon balm. These herbs appear to be safe although some, such as valerian, should not be taken with other medications or used routinely.

When herbal supplements became more popular in the United States it didn't take long for them to find their way into weight-loss products.

Many health professionals worry that consumers don't have enough information to make good decisions about herbal weight-loss products. "Herbal" does not mean that a product is safe.

Herbal Weight-Loss Products

The "herbal" in herbal weight-loss products could refer to several compounds, but in many cases it refers to the addition of ma huang (ephedra). The discussion about ephedra-containing weight-loss products can sometimes be confusing because terms that are technically different are sometimes used interchangeably. The first step is to understand the terms *ephedra, ephedrine alkaloids,* and *ephedrine.* Ephedra is a botanical term that refers to a plant genus. Some species of ephedra contain ephedrine alkaloids in their stems and branches. Ephedrine is one example of an ephedrine alkaloid. In traditional Chinese medicine, ma huang is extracted from the stems and branches of *Ephedra sinica* Stapf, a species of the plant genus ephedra. Six different ephedrine alkaloids are found in the stems and branches of the ma huang; of the six, ephedrine is the main active ingredient. In addition to being extracted from plants, ephedrine may be synthesized in the laboratory.

Although there is a distinction between the terms, in everyday language *ephedra* is generally used to refer to both herbal and nonherbal dietary supplements that contain ephedrine. Many herbal supplements list the source of ephedrine as ma huang, so the term *ephedra* or *ephedrine* does not appear on the label. Just because it doesn't say *ephedra* or *ephedrine* doesn't mean that ephedrine is not present.

Ma huang is used in traditional Chinese medicine to treat asthma and nasal congestion but not to promote weight loss. Ephedrine is added to over-the-counter medications in the United States as a decongestant, which is consistent with the traditional use by Chinese herbalists. Ma huang (ephedrine) is also found in dietary supplements sold to promote weight loss and to increase energy. The use of ma huang to stimulate weight loss is an American twist on the use of a traditional Chinese medicine.

Ephedrine-containing dietary supplements may also contain caffeine. Caffeine contains the active ingredient methylxanthine, a compound known to enhance the weight-loss effect of ephedrine. In herbal dietary supplements the source of the caffeine may be guarana or kola nuts. Regardless of the source, check to see whether the dietary supplement being sold for weight loss or to increase energy contains a source of ephedrine or a source of caffeine. Remember that the words *ephedra* or *caffeine* may not appear on the label.

The safety of ephedrine-containing dietary supplements (with or without caffeine) is hotly debated. The most contentious issue is dose. Scientists simply do not agree on the level of ephedrine that is considered safe. The FDA has proposed that not more than 8 milligrams of ephedrine alkaloids be used in a 6-hour period or not more than 24 milligrams in a 24-hour period. The FDA would also like to require a statement that warns people not to take an ephedrine-containing product for more than seven days. However, not all experts agree with the proposed FDA guidelines. They contend that a single dose should not contain more than 30 milligrams of ephedrine alkaloids and that up to 90 milligrams of ephedrine alkaloids in a 24-hour period is safe. Regarding long-term use, these scientists suggest that the recommended dose be consumed for not more than six months. The disagreement among scientists has made it difficult for consumers to judge safety.

Unfortunately, there is a lack of scientific studies to establish a safe dose for ephedrine. Part of the FDA concern is based on the information obtained from the FDA adverse events reports (AER). Any person who has experienced an adverse event caused by a dietary supplement can report the experience to the FDA by calling 1-800-FDA-1088 or via the Internet at www.fda.gov/medwatch/report/hcp.htm. In 1997 the FDA became alarmed because more than 800 adverse events involving ephedra-containing dietary supplements were reported. These 800 reports accounted for 50 to 60% of all the AER that the FDA received. The adverse events included insomnia, increased heart rate, increased blood pressure, and headaches, where were not surprising because these are well-known side effects. However, there were some reported deaths in otherwise healthy young or middle-aged people, which were both surprising and tragic.

The problem with the AER system is that information obtained from self-reported adverse effects is not the same as information obtained from scientific studies. Unfortunately, many of the AER are not detailed and do not include the amount of ephedrine or ephedrine alkaloids that were consumed. Because dose is an important issue, not knowing the exact dosage taken makes interpreting the AER almost impossible. Also, many of the ephedrine-containing dietary supplements contain other ingredients (such as caffeine), and it is not known whether the adverse effects are due to the ephedrine by itself or in combination with other compounds. Everyone agrees that more information is needed. That leaves consumers who wish to take ephedrine-containing dietary supplements in the position of deciding what is a safe dose. The more conservative approach is to apply the proposed FDA guidelines. But the questions don't stop once you have decided on a safety guideline. A tricky issue related to an ephedrine-containing dietary supplement is knowing the amount of active ingredient actually contained in the dietary supplement that you buy. The amount of ephedrine or ephedrine alkaloids that is extracted from the stems and leaves of the *Ephedra* species varies with the growing conditions and the method of extraction. If amounts are not standardized, then the ephedrine in a supplement can be very different when compared to another brand or even a different batch of the same brand. One of the greatest dangers to consumers is the lack of standardization of ephedrine-containing dietary supplements.

Once you have determined whether the ephedrine-containing dietary supplement is safe, you must answer questions about effectiveness. Ephedrine in combination with caffeine is being studied to determine its ability to produce short-term weight loss. Caffeine enhances the action of ephedrine, so the ephedrine and caffeine combination is more effective than either compound alone. At the present time studies show that the use of ephedrine and caffeine by obese people could produce a short-term weight loss of 8 to 9 pounds. An important point is that the studies have been conducted on obese subjects (usually with a BMI greater than 35), not on non-obese subjects. Also be aware that the increased energy that such a supplement produces is likely due to the stimulant effects of both the ephedrine (remarkably similar in chemical structure to amphetamine) and caffeine.

Herbal supplements are widely available, but they are minimally regulated. The act that allows this is the Dietary Supplement Health and Education Act. Keep in mind that *you* are the one who needs to be educated about dietary supplements and that *you* must look out for your own health.

Eat Well and Supplement Wisely

This portion of the book has covered some of the dietary supplements currently on the market. It could never cover all the dietary supplements available because the market changes so rapidly. So does the body of scientific research. That means that a supplement that is on the market today may be found to be unsafe or ineffective in the future. On the other hand, a supplement whose safety or effectiveness today is questionable may be shown to be both safe and effective in the future. Because your health is one of the most important parts of your life, you should become a lifelong open-minded skeptic about which supplements to choose.

Never underestimate the connection between food and health. At present there is a strong case for getting nutrients from a variety of foods. There is an even stronger case for being physically active daily. Make diet and exercise the foundation of your good health habits and then consider the role that supplements might play. To make the best decisions, you need to thoroughly evaluate the most current information available and match it to your individual needs.

It may seem quicker, and perhaps easier, if this book simply gave you a diet to follow. But a diet is a pattern of eating, and a pattern needs to be more flexible and individualized than a predetermined eating plan. This book presents nutrition information and a logical approach to applying that information. It is designed for people who want to focus on good nutrition as part of a healthy lifestyle, but these things take both time and effort. Food first, supplements second is a philosophy that will serve you well.

THE BIG EASY
(TIPS THAT TAKE VIRTUALLY NO EFFORT)

✔ Buy nutritious foods when you stop to fill your car with gas. Most gas stations carry orange juice, bottled water, some fresh fruit (usually apples, bananas, and oranges), bagels, small bags of nuts, and small packages of Fig Newtons.

✔ Pick up a deli dinner on the way home from work. Order sandwiches on whole-grain bread, choose lean meats, ask for lots of vegetable toppings, and add a bean or marinated vegetable salad as a side dish.

✔ Buy fresh produce that has been cleaned and prepared. A variety of packaged salads are available; choose the ones that have the darkest green lettuce. Add oil and vinegar to a packaged cole slaw mix for a quick, easy, and healthful side dish. And what could be easier than the small packages of peeled carrots?

✔ Most dried fruit is now available in resealable bags. Dried plums (very sweet!), mixed fruits, raisins, and apricots are good snack foods to keep in your desk or backpack.

✔ Unsweetened applesauce comes in small cups and can be stored on the shelf at room temperature.

✔ Try some higher-fiber grain dishes. Couscous, which is made from durum wheat, can be added to boiling water and is ready after 5 minutes of soaking. Cracked bulgur wheat takes 15 minutes to cook. Wheat and lentil pilafs take the same time as rice to cook.

✔ Incorporate beans, lentils, and split peas into your diet by buying canned or dehydrated beans, bean soups, and chili. All that you need to do is to heat them or add boiling water.

✔ Whole-wheat frozen waffles are a quick and easy breakfast meal. Toast them, break in half, spoon on yogurt, and eat them as you would eat a sandwich.

✔ Plain microwave popcorn is a snack that's easy to fix, involves no clean-up, and is high in fiber.

✔ More precooked red meat and poultry are available. Sliced chicken and turkey breasts are available precooked and can be heated in the microwave or conventional oven, sometimes in the packages that they come in.

✔ Buy frozen "healthy meals." Stouffer's Lean Cuisine, Healthy Choice, and other companies sell a variety of meals that have reasonably sized portions that meet healthy nutritional guidelines.

TIME AND
MONEY

Consumers must balance time and money concerns when deciding which foods to purchase. Healthy foods, such as fresh fruits and vegetables, often take time to prepare. Prepared foods are convenient but are higher priced because of the cost of the labor involved in preparation. If you see a healthy food that you would like to buy but are put off by the price, remember there is usually a low cost alternative—buy the ingredients and put in the labor. If you are willing to spend your money, rather than your time, on food, take advantage of the healthy foods that are prepared.

If you have more money than time:	If you have more time than money:
Buy prepared salad greens or spinach in a bag.	Buy lettuce and spinach, wash it, tear it, and store it in a plastic bag. Eat three salads for the price of one prepared salad.
Buy the "gourmet" greens that feature a mix of lesser-known dark leafy salad greens.	Buy a package of mixed lettuce seeds and plant in the garden. Thin the lettuce and tear off the outside leaves and use in salads.
Buy a veggie tray (carrots, cauliflower, broccoli) or prepared vegetables in a bag.	Have a friend buy veggies at a farmer's market or roadside stand, and clean and cut them for both of you.
Buy fresh fruits that have been prepared, such as cut melons or cubed fruit salad.	Offer to pick a friend or neighbor's tomatoes or fruit trees.
Buy freshly squeezed orange juice.	Buy frozen orange juice and reconstitute.
Buy instant oatmeal in packages and add boiling water.	Buy a large container of oatmeal and cook (takes 5 minutes to cook plus clean up).
Buy three-bean salad at a deli.	Make your own three-bean salad.
Buy food in individual serving containers (such as cottage cheese and fruit).	Pack your own lunch and save by buying larger containers of the same food and packing it in reusable plastic containers.
Buy healthy frozen meals (usually low-fat, moderate protein, lots of vegetables and other carbohydrates).	Use the meals as a menu guideline but prepare the foods yourself (usually cheaper if self-prepared).

BEYOND THE BORDERS
(TRY A NEW FOOD—YOU MAY LIKE IT)

Before the days of easy travel and mass transportation of food products, each region of the world developed its cuisine based on products that were locally grown. These traditional diets, often known as ethnic cuisine, are sometimes very different from the diet on which you've been raised. Because people around the world need the same nutrients, it is not surprising that a closer look at traditional ethnic foods may yield some different ways to obtain a particular nutrient. It can't hurt to try something new; you may find that you like it.

Whole-Grain Carbohydrates

Whole grains play an important role in chronic disease prevention. They provide carbohydrates and many of the nutrients that are lacking in the U.S. diet: fiber, B vitamins, vitamin E, selenium, zinc, copper, and magnesium.

WHOLE-GRAIN CARBOHYDRATES

Food	Description and use
Buckwheat (kasha, groats)	The seed of a plant related to rhubarb. Neither a wheat nor a grain, buckwheat contains approximately the same nutrients as whole grains. Kasha (groats) is roasted buckwheat eaten as a cooked breakfast cereal or added to pasta.
Bulgur (bulghur)	A wheat berry with a nutty flavor. Best known as part of the cold Middle Eastern salad tabbouleh.
Cornmeal (stone ground)	Stone-ground cornmeal (which includes the oily germ and must be refrigerated) is made by grinding dried corn. Most cornmeal sold in the United States is degerminated and does not require refrigeration. However, the degermination process removes most of the fiber and many of the minerals.
Cracked wheat	A wheat berry that has been cracked to produce smaller particles. Used as an ingredient in some whole-wheat breads.
Quinoa	Pronounced *keen-wa*. High-protein grain of the Inca, cooked and eaten the same as bulgur or rice.

Beans and Legumes

Beans and legumes, in general, are high-carbohydrate, high-fiber, moderate-protein, low-fat foods that contain a variety of nutrients, particularly iron. You may be surprised that there are so many choices. See the charts on pages 165-167.

Soy

Soybeans are also legumes, but they are listed separately because they contain isoflavones and more calcium and fat than other legumes. Soy products are often high in sodium. Soy foods are now widely available in U.S. supermarkets. Some soy foods and their notable nutrients are listed on pages 168-169.

Protein From Meats

In the United States the term *meat* often refers to beef, lamb and pork, but there are some other lean meat sources that you may want to consider. Native Americans and Alaskan natives have eaten many of these for years. The following are excellent low-fat meat sources of protein, iron, and zinc.

Roasted buffalo
Roasted elk
Roasted moose
Roasted rabbit
Roasted venison (deer meat)

Fish, Nuts, and Seeds

Fish, nuts, seeds, and vegetable oils are the preferred sources of fat over animal fats. Olive oil and canola oil are high in monounsaturated fats (fats that are thought to be heart healthy). Walnuts and wheat germ are high in omega-3 fatty acids, a polyunsaturated heart-healthy fat. The following fish also contain a lot of omega-3 fatty acids and would be good choices to add to your diet.

Anchovies
Bluefish (blue runner)
Herring
Mackerel (ono, Atlantic mackerel, king mackerel, and Spanish mackerel)
Sablefish (known as Alaska cod and black cod, but it is not a true cod)
Salmon
Sardines (sardines are young herrings packed in oil, water, pesto, hot sauce, or mustard)
Tuna (albacore, bluefin, bonito, skipjack, and yellowfin)

Exotic Fruits and Vegetables

Take some time to study the produce section of your local supermarket, stop at a small ethnic market, or explore the offerings at a farmer's market and you will be surprised at the variety of fruits and vegetables available. The charts on pages 170-173 describe lesser-known fruits and vegetables. Some are excellent sources of vitamins A or C, but all fruits and vegetables provide some phytochemicals, small amounts of many nutrients, and a variety of tastes and textures. In some cases the amount normally eaten is small; thus, the amount of nutrients is low but still a contribution to the overall dietary intake.

Calcium

Consider these high-calcium sources that have approximately the same amount of calcium as an 8-ounce glass of milk (300 milligrams of calcium):

1 ounce whole-roasted sesame seeds (280 milligrams)

6 whole sardines (275 milligrams)

80 grams (or ⅕ block) of tofu processed with calcium sulfate (260 milligrams)

8-ounce glass of calcium-fortified soy milk (300-400 milligrams)

8-ounce glass of calcium-fortified orange juice (350 milligrams)

8-ounce glass of calcium-fortified rice beverage (300 milligrams) [Note that rice beverages do not have the same amount of protein as soy milk or cow's milk.]

Iron

Consider these high-iron sources if you are having trouble getting enough iron in your diet (premenopausal women need 18 milligrams daily):

3 ounces canned clams (24 milligrams)

3 ounces oysters (7.8 milligrams)

1 ounce whole-roasted sesame seeds (4.2 milligrams)

A Note About Seaweed

Calcium and iron are two nutrients that are often deficient in women's diets. Dairy products are exceptionally rich in calcium but are poor sources of iron. Meats are an excellent source of iron but are poor sources of calcium. Seaweed (depending on the type) can be a good source of both minerals. For example, 10 grams (2$^1/_2$ tablespoons) of hizikia fusiforme (hijiki) contain 150 milligrams of calcium and 5.4 milligrams of iron. Seaweed can be soaked and added to stir-fry or used as an ingredient in soup.

BEANS AND LEGUMES

Food	Description and use	Notable nutrients (in $^{1}/_{2}$-cup serving)
Black and calypso beans	A flavorful bean that can be highly seasoned. Widely used in the Caribbean, Brazil, and Mexico.	Protein: 8 grams Carbohydrate: 20 grams Fiber: 7 grams Iron: 1.81 milligrams
Black-eyed peas (cow peas) and pigeon peas (gandules or gungo beans)	Black-eyed peas are a small bean native to China, used in southern U.S. cooking as well. Pigeon peas are used in Caribbean dishes.	Protein: 7 grams Carbohydrate: 18 grams Fiber: 6 grams Iron: 2.16 milligrams
Fava beans (broad beans)	Large kidney-shaped bean used in Mediterranean cooking. They have a slightly bitter taste compared to other beans. *Note: Some people of Mediterranean descent cannot digest fava beans and should not eat them.*	Protein: 6 grams Carbohydrate: 14 grams Fiber: 4.5 grams Iron: 1.13 milligrams
Garbanzo beans (chickpeas, ceci beans)	Bean used in Mediterranean cooking. Firm even when cooked. Hummus is a roasted garbanzo-bean dip. Falafel is made from ground chick peas and fried.	Protein: 7 grams Carbohydrate: 23 grams Fiber: 6 grams Iron: 2.37 milligrams

Kidney beans:
    Anasazi beans
    Appaloosa beans
    Cannellini beans
    Cranberry beans
    European soldier beans
    Jackson wonder beans
    Great northern beans
    Pink beans
    Pinto beans
	There are many kinds of kidney beans. Any of these dried beans should be soaked and then cooked for about 40 to 60 minutes. Most are available canned but will be softer in texture. Used in a variety of dishes including stew, soup, and chili and in combination with rice.	Protein: 6.5 grams
		Carbohydrate: 20 grams
		Fiber: 8 grams
		Iron: 1.61 milligrams

BEANS AND LEGUMES (CONTINUED)

Food	Description and use	Notable nutrients (in $^1/_2$-cup serving)
Kidney beans (continued): Rattlesnake beans Red (white) kidney beans Scarlet runner beans Swedish brown beans Tongues-of-fire beans Trout beans	There are many kinds of kidney beans. Any of these dried beans should be soaked and then cooked for about 40 to 60 minutes. Most are available canned but will be softer in texture. Used in a variety of dishes including stew, soup, and chili and in combination with rice.	Protein: 6.5 grams Carbohydrate: 20 grams Fiber: 8 grams Iron: 1.61 milligrams
Lentils Dals (dahls)	Dal is a Hindi word for dried peas, beans, and lentils. Lentils require no soaking and cook in less than 30 minutes. Used in soups and salads.	Protein: 9 grams Carbohydrate: 20 grams Fiber: 8 grams Iron: 3.29 milligrams
Lima beans and Christmas limas	One of the few beans available frozen and eaten as a vegetable. Also used in salads, soups, and stews.	Protein: 3.5 grams Carbohydrate: 10 grams Fiber: 3.5 grams Iron: 1.12 milligrams
Mung beans	Slightly sweet-flavored bean used in China and India. Also used for bean sprouts.	Protein: 7 grams Carbohydrate: 19 grams Fiber: 8 grams Iron: 1.41 milligrams
Navy beans: French navy beans Steuben yellow-eyed beans	In the United States traditionally served as baked beans.	Protein: 8 grams Carbohydrate: 24 grams Fiber: 6 grams Iron: 2.25 milligrams

BEANS AND LEGUMES (CONTINUED)

Food	Description and use	Notable nutrients (in 1/2-cup serving)
Split peas (green and yellow)	Require no soaking and become mushy when cooked; thus, they're perfect for soup. Green split peas are more flavorful than yellow split peas.	Protein: 8 grams Carbohydrate: 21 grams Fiber: 8 grams Iron: 1.26 milligrams
Tepary beans	Similar to pinto beans and used in southwestern United States and in Mexico.	Protein: 7 grams Carbohydrate: 22 grams Fiber: 7 grams Iron: 2.22 milligrams
Winged beans (goas)	Tropical legumes with a flavor similar to a cranberry bean but the texture of starchy green beans. Higher in fat, calcium, and iron than most beans and contain no fiber.	Protein: 9 grams Carbohydrate: 13 grams Fat: 5 grams Fiber: 0 grams Iron: 3.7 milligrams Calcium: 122 milligrams

SOY

Food	Description and use	Notable nutrients (in ¹/₂-cup serving)
Fresh soybeans	Can be purchased fresh or frozen in the pod and cooked in boiling water.	Protein: 10 grams Carbohydrate: 8 grams Fat: 5 grams Fiber: 5 grams Iron: 2.7 milligrams Calcium: 60 milligrams
Dried soybeans	Can be soaked, cooked, and eaten in a manner similar to other beans; however, they are more often used to make curds and milks.	Protein: 15 grams Carbohydrate: 9 grams Fat: 8 grams Fiber: 5 grams Iron: 4.42 milligrams Calcium: 88 milligrams
Dried, roasted soybeans	Eaten as a snack.	Protein: 34 grams Carbohydrate: 28 grams Fat: 19 grams Fiber: 7 grams Iron: 3.4 milligrams Calcium: 120 milligrams
Soy milk	Liquid obtained from pressing ground, cooked soybeans. Available as full-fat, low-fat, and nonfat. Often calcium fortified.	If fortified: Protein: 3 grams Carbohydrate: 11 grams Fat: varies 0-2.5 grams Fiber: .5 grams Iron: .72 milligrams Calcium: 200 milligrams

SOY (CONTINUED)

Food	Description and use	Notable nutrients (in ¹/₂-cup serving)
Tempeh	Fermented soybean cake.	Protein: 16 grams Carbohydrate: 14 grams Fat: 6 grams Fiber: 0 grams Iron: 1.91 milligrams Calcium: 77 milligrams
Tofu (comes as extra-firm, firm, regular, or soft)	Nutrient content varies depending on firmness and process (if calcium sulfate is used then calcium content is significant, as shown in nutrient column).	Protein: 8 grams Carbohydrate: 2 grams Fat: 5 grams Fiber: less than 1 gram Iron: 1.38 milligrams Calcium: 138 milligrams

EXOTIC FRUITS

Fruit	Description	Notable nutrients
Papaya	Large, orange-pulped sweet or astringent fruit with peppery black seeds.	Vitamin A and C, calcium
Mango	Sweet, orange-fleshed tropical fruit.	Vitamin A and C
Persimmon	American and Japanese varieties vary in shape and size, but both are sweet when ripe.	Vitamin A and C
Feijoa	South American fruit with a pineapple guava taste.	Vitamin C
Guava	Sweet tropical fruit.	Vitamin C
Kiwi	Fuzzy brown fruit with green pulp and black seeds with a sweet and tart flavor.	Vitamin C
Litchi	Asian fruit with the flavor of muscat grapes. Available fresh or canned.	Vitamin C
Mandarin oranges (mikan)	Easily peeled citrus fruit with a sweet orange flavor.	Vitamin C
Carambola (star fruit)	Native to Asia, sweet to tart flavor used in chutneys and sweet and sour dishes.	Vitamin A
Loquat	Japanese plum with a sour cherry flavor.	Vitamin A
Mamey	Large West Indian fruit with an apricot flavor.	Vitamin A
Passion fruit (granadilla)	Sweet and sour tropical fruit generally used for sauces and beverages.	Vitamin A
Zapote (sapodilla)	Member of the persimmon family with a brown sugar flavor.	Vitamin A

EXOTIC FRUITS (CONTINUED)

Fruit	Description
Acerola cherries	Acidic fruit of Native Americans and West Indians eaten fresh or made into jam.
Akee (genipa)	Cherry-sized tropical fruit that tastes like a grape.
Asian pear	Juicy, crunchy fruit with an apple and pear flavor.
Breadfruit	Related to the fig family. Bland flavor with a texture like fresh bread.
Buffalo berry	Wild berry used by native Americans in a sauce for buffalo meat. Acidic flavor.
Cactus (prickly pear)	Purple-red pear-shaped fruit of a specific species of cactus.
Cherimoya (custard apple)	Tropical fruit with a custard-like texture and mango and strawberry flavor.
Chinese date (jujube)	Similar in taste and use to a prune.
Durian (Malaysian cantaloupe)	Custard-like texture and a sweet flavor but foul smell.
Kumquat	Small citrus fruit with thin rind. Eaten whole for a burst of sweet and sour flavor.
Naranjilla	Sweet and sour fruit native to South America.
Papaw	Fruit of Native Americans with a banana and pear flavor and custard-like texture.
Rambutan	Native to Malaysia and similar to a litchi but with a more acidic and almond flavor.
Ugli fruit	Hybrid citrus from Jamaica similar in taste to a mandarin orange.

EXOTIC VEGETABLES

Vegetable	Description	Notable Nutrients
Fennel	Root vegetable with mild licorice taste.	Vitamin A and C, calcium
Greens (chard, collard, dandelion greens, kale, milkweed, mustard greens, pokeweed, purslane)	Greens with stronger flavors than traditional salad greens. May be eaten raw or cooked.	Vitamin A and C, calcium
Amaranth (can also be ground into a flour)	Green- or purple-leafed vegetable used like spinach in Chinese and Caribbean cooking.	Vitamin A and C
Bok choy	Mild-tasting Chinese cabbage, eaten raw, pickled, or cooked.	Vitamin A and C
Napa cabbage	Very mild, crinkle-leafed Chinese snow cabbage.	Vitamin A and C
Kohlrabi	Cabbage and turnip hybrid that forms a bulb and is cooked like a root vegetable.	Vitamin C Cruciferous vegetable
Okra	Asparagus flavor. Gelatinous when cooked for a long time. Used in soups and stews as a thickener.	Vitamin C
Cardoon	Closely related to an artichoke.	Vitamin A
Chayote	Central American squash-like vegetable.	Vitamin A
Plantain	Known as a cooking banana for its squash flavor when cooked. Starchy.	Vitamin A

EXOTIC VEGETABLES (CONTINUED)

Vegetable	Description
Arugula	Salad green known for its strong, peppery taste.
Bitter melon	A vegetable (not a melon) that looks like a bumpy cucumber and tastes like a squash.
Burdock root (gobo)	A root vegetable used in Japanese diets as a flavor accent.
Celery root (celeriac)	Root vegetable from a specially bred celery plant, eaten raw or cooked.
Daikon	Strong-flavored white radish native to Asia, eaten raw or cooked.
Fuzzy melon	Chinese squash (not a melon) with a bland flavor.
Long beans (Chinese green beans, yardlong beans)	Very long and thin green beans.
Radicchio	A variety of chicory used in salads and known for its biting flavor.
Sorrel	Tart-flavored leaf used in salads or cooked as a vegetable.
Tomatillo	Mexican green tomato used in sauces. Does not have nutrient content of red tomatoes.
Winter melon	Zucchini flavor.

IF YOU NEED MORE OF A NUTRIENT, TRY THESE FOODS

Nutrient	Food Sources
Fiber, carbohydrates, and whole grains	Bran or other high fiber cereals Whole-grain breads Brown rice Whole-wheat noodles Sesame seeds Nuts Wheat germ Lentils, split peas, dried beans
Protein	Fish (broiled) Soy products Nonfat or low-fat milk Lean meat or poultry (small portions not fried) Beans, lentils, split peas Nuts
Fats	Olive oil Canola oil Fish Nuts Seeds Soybeans
Vitamin E	Vegetable oil Oil-based salad dressing, such as Italian Soybeans Almonds and other nuts Sunflower seeds Wheat germ
Vitamin C	Orange juice Grapefruit juice Cantaloupe Green or red peppers Broccoli Cabbage (raw)
Vitamin A	Carrots Spinach Tomatoes Broccoli Apricots Cantaloupe
Calcium	Nonfat or low-fat milk Cheese Cottage cheese Kefir Yogurt Frozen yogurt Leafy green vegetables
Iron	Clams Fish Meat Poultry Dried beans Tofu Whole-grain breads and cereals Leafy green vegetables

Nutrient	Food Sources
Thiamin	Whole-grain breads and cereals Dried beans Pork
Riboflavin	Nonfat or low-fat milk Leafy green vegetables Whole-grain breads and cereals
Niacin	Fish Poultry Meat Eggs Nonfat or low-fat milk Whole grain breads and cereals Nuts
Magnesium	Oysters Dried beans Whole-grain breads and cereals Soy milk Milk Yogurt Potatoes
Potassium	Fish Milk Dried beans Many fruits, particularly banana Many vegetables Potato
Zinc	Whole-grain breads and cereals Nuts Seeds Dried beans Fish Soybeans Nonfat or low-fat milk Yogurt
Vitamin B_6	Whole-grain breads and cereals Dried beans Leafy green vegetables Bananas Fish Meat Poultry
Folate	Leafy green vegetables Whole-grain breads and cereals Dried beans Orange juice

FUNCTIONAL FOODS, DESIGNER FOODS, AND NUTRACEUTICALS

Functional and designer foods are conventional foods that have nutrients added to protect against chronic disease. Nutraceuticals are nutrients found in food (or supplements) that may have a medicinal effect. The following are some examples of these foods.

Margarine with added plant sterols and plant stanols (chemically similar to cholesterol and therefore able to keep cholesterol from being absorbed)
Omega-3 fatty acid–enriched eggs (not available in all states)
Probiotics (live microbial food supplement, such as *Lactobacillus* or *Bifidobacterium,* added to a product)
Acidophilus milk
Buttermilk
Fermented vegetables
Kefir or koumiss
Yogurt

The following products are controversial because of a lack of scientific evidence of their benefits.

Beverages with the antioxidant vitamins E and C added
Beverages with herbs added (such as echinacea, ginkgo, kava, ginseng, and saw palmetto)
Soups with herbs added (such as echinacea or St. John's wort)
Tomato products with added lycopene
Medicinal food bars (with added nutrients such as L-arginine)

HOW TO INTERPRET THE NUMBERS
ON FOOD LABELS

Once people learn about Dietary Reference Intakes (DRI), they have an idea of how much of a nutrient they need to consume daily. They often go to the grocery store and look at food labels expecting to find the DRI. Instead they find a new term, Daily Values (DV). So why isn't the DRI on a food label? The reason is that Dietary Reference Intakes vary according to age and gender. For example, if you are 30 years old you need 1,000 milligrams of calcium per day, but if you are 60 years old you need 1,200 milligrams daily. The label, because it lists percentages, can only be based on one figure. In the case of calcium, the figure used for label calculations is 1,000 milligrams. The Daily Values are a good estimate of the amount of a nutrient you need. Daily Values are not as specific for your age and gender as the Dietary Reference Intakes.

There are no Daily Values established for sugars or protein. Daily Values are listed on the label both as a number (grams or milligrams) and as a percentage for total fat, saturated fat, cholesterol, sodium, total carbohydrate, and dietary fiber. Other nutrients are listed on the food label but only with % DV. The following chart represents 100% of the Daily Value for the nutrients listed. (Note: Not all nutrients that have a DV are listed.)

DAILY VALUES USED FOR FOOD LABEL CALCULATIONS

Nutrient	100% Daily Value	Nutrient	100% Daily Value
Vitamin A	900 RE (5,000 IU)	Calcium	1000 mg
Vitamin D	10 mcg (400 IU)	Iron	18 mg
Vitamin E	20 mg (30 IU)	Zinc	15 mg
Vitamin C	60 mg	Magnesium	400 mg
Thiamin	1.5 mg	Potassium	3500 mg
Riboflavin	1.7 mg	Iodine	150 mcg
Niacin	20 mg	Copper	2 mg
Vitamin B_6	2 mg	Chromium	120 mcg
Folate	400 mcg	Selenium	70 mcg
Vitamin B_{12}	6 mcg	Manganese	2 mg

CALL IN THE
ACRONYM POLICE

Consumers often are confused because there are so many different nutrition terms, and nearly all of them are abbreviated. Help! Call in the acronym police! The following list briefly describes the most commonly used terms.

Dietary Reference Intakes (DRI). Dietary Reference Intakes are the newest standard used to assess nutrient intake in healthy people. The DRI helps to answer the question, "How much of each nutrient do I need?" The DRI is made up of four values: the EAR, RDA, AI, and UL (see the following list).

Estimated Average Requirement (EAR): The EAR is a median value. For half of the healthy population, this value would cover their need for that nutrient. For the other half of the healthy population, this value would be inadequate.

Recommended Dietary Allowances (RDA): The average level of a nutrient that would meet the needs of about 97% of the healthy population. The RDA represents a "recommended intake" even though it exceeds the dietary needs for many people.

Adequate Intake (AI): An approximation of the level of a nutrient that would be adequate. Used when scientific data are not complete enough to establish an EAR.

Tolerable Upper Intake Level (UL): The highest average daily intake of a nutrient that would not likely pose a risk.

Since the 1940s the RDA has been the standard used to judge the nutrient adequacy of a diet. Now the standard is the Dietary Reference Intakes (DRI). The RDA has not been lost but it is now part of a better standard. The confusing part is that the DRI were introduced in stages beginning in 1997. While the DRI were being phased in, some nutrients had a DRI while other nutrients had an RDA. DRI have now been released for all vitamins and minerals.

Daily Values (DV). Daily Values are the nutrient standard used on the food label. They reflect the nutrient needs of the "average" person consuming 2,000 to 2,500 calories daily. They are best used to compare the amount of a nutrient in a food. For example, if you are comparing two cans of soup, the one with the higher percentage of DV has more of that nutrient.

FOOD
LABEL

Nutrition Facts

Serving size 1/4 cup (45 g)
Servings per package 8

Amount per serving

Calories 150   Calories from Fat 10

	% Daily Value*
Total Fat 1.5 g	2%
Saturated Fat 0 g	0%
Cholesterol 0 mg	0%
Sodium 0 mg	0%
Total Carbohydrate 35 g	12%
Dietary fiber 3 g	12%
Sugars 0 g	0%
Protein 4 g	

Vitamin A	0%
Vitamin C	0%
Calcium	0%
Iron	2%

Percent Daily Values are based on a 2,000 calorie diet. Your daily values may be higher or lower depending on your calorie needs.

	Calories	2,000	2,500
Total Fat	Less than	65 g	80 g
Sat Fat	Less than	20 g	25 g
Cholesterol	Less than	300 mg	300 mg
Total Carbohydrate		300 g	375g
Dietary fiber		25 g	30 g

Calories per gram: Fat 9 • Carbohydrate 4 • Protein 4

Ingredients: Long grain brown rice, sweet brown rice, wild rice bits

SUPPLEMENT
LABEL

Supplement Facts

Serving size 1 capsule

Amount per serving	% Daily Value*
Vitamin E 400 IU	1333%

Garlic 200 mg	*
Lutein 6 mg	*

* Daily Value not established

Ingredients: di-alpha tocopheryl acetate, garlic, lutein, gelatin, glycerin, polysorbate 80.

Storage: Keep in a cool dry place, tightly closed.

Suggested Use: One (1) capsule daily with a meal

Keep out of the reach of children
Expiration date: Dec 2004

HEALTHY WAYS VITAMINS, INC.
LONG BEACH, CA 90805

HOW TO CONVERT INTERNATIONAL UNITS (IU)
TO CURRENTLY USED MEASURES

Vitamin A. To convert IU to micrograms (mcg) RE (retinol equivalents), determine whether the food is of animal or plant origin. For animal sources divide IU by 3.33; for plant sources divide by 10. For example, a supplement contains 100 IU of beta-carotene. Beta-carotene is derived from plant sources. Divide 100 IU by 10. The 100 IU of beta-carotene = 10 micrograms (mcg) RE of vitamin A.

Vitamin D. To convert IU to micrograms of vitamin D, divide IU by 40. For example, a supplement contains 1,000 IU of vitamin D. Divide 1,000 by 40; 1,000 IU = 25 micrograms of vitamin D.

Vitamin E. To convert IU to milligrams (mg) of alpha-tocopherol, divide by 1.5. For example, a supplement contains 300 IU of vitamin E. Divide 300 by 1.5; 300 IU = 200 milligrams of vitamin E.

BODY MASS INDEX (BMI)

	18	19	20	21	22	23	24	25	26	27	28	29	30	31	32	33	34	35	36	37	38
4'10"	86	91	96	100	105	110	115	119	124	129	134	138	143	148	153	158	162	167	172	177	181
4'11"	89	94	99	104	109	114	119	124	128	133	138	143	148	153	158	163	168	173	178	183	188
5'0"	92	97	102	107	112	118	123	128	133	138	143	148	153	158	163	168	174	179	184	189	194
5'1"	95	100	106	111	116	122	127	132	137	143	148	153	158	164	169	174	180	185	190	195	201
5'2"	98	104	109	115	120	126	131	136	142	147	153	158	164	169	175	180	186	191	196	202	207
5'3"	102	107	113	118	124	130	135	141	146	152	158	163	169	174	180	186	191	197	203	208	214
5'4"	105	110	116	122	128	134	140	145	151	157	163	169	174	180	186	192	197	204	209	215	221
5'5"	108	114	120	126	132	138	144	150	156	162	168	174	180	186	192	198	204	210	216	222	228
5'6"	112	118	124	130	136	142	148	155	161	167	173	179	186	192	198	204	210	216	223	229	235
5'7"	115	121	127	134	140	146	153	159	166	172	178	185	191	198	204	211	217	223	230	236	242
5'8"	118	125	131	138	144	151	158	164	171	177	184	190	197	203	210	216	223	230	236	243	249
5'9"	122	128	135	142	149	155	162	169	176	182	189	196	203	209	216	223	230	236	243	250	257
5'10"	126	132	139	146	153	160	167	174	181	188	195	202	209	216	222	229	236	243	250	257	264
5'11"	129	136	143	150	157	165	172	179	186	193	200	208	215	222	229	236	243	250	257	265	272
6'0"	132	140	147	154	162	169	177	184	191	199	206	213	221	228	235	242	250	258	265	272	279
6'1"	136	144	151	159	166	174	182	189	197	204	212	219	227	235	242	250	257	265	272	280	288
6'2"	141	148	155	163	171	179	186	194	202	210	218	225	233	241	249	256	264	272	280	287	295
6'3"	144	152	160	168	176	184	192	200	208	216	224	232	240	248	256	264	272	279	287	295	303
6'4"	148	156	164	172	180	189	197	205	213	221	230	238	246	254	263	271	279	287	295	304	312

How to use this table: Find your height in the first column. In that row, find your approximate weight. The number at the top of the column where your weight appears is your BMI.

ANNA'S COMPLETE NUTRIENT ANALYSIS

	Fiber (g)	CHO (g)	Protein (g)	Fat (g)	Vitamin E (mg)	Vitamin C (mg)	Vitamin A (mcg RE)	Calcium (mg)	Iron (mg)	Thiamin (mg)	Riboflavin (mg)	Niacin (mg)	Cholesterol (mg)	Magnesium (mg)	Potassium (mg)	Sodium (mg)	Zinc (mg)	Vitamin B6 (mg)	Folate (mcg)
2 slices whole-grain toast	4	24	6	2	0.32	0	0	48	1.8	0.22	0.18	2.28	0	28	106	254	0.66	0.18	21
1 poached egg	0	1	6	5	0.52	0	95	24	0.72	0.02	0.21	0.03	212	5	60	140	0.55	0.06	17
1 cup grapefruit juice	0	22	1	<1	0.12	72	2	17	0.49	0.1	0.05	0.57	0	25	378	2	0.22	0.05	72
1 cup black tea	0	1	0	0	0	0	0	0	.05	0	0	.03	0	7	88	7	.05	0	12
1 cup split pea soup	3	21	7	1	0.13	0	5	20	0.94	.19	0.05	.87	0	17	355	233	.49	0.02	32
3½-inch bagel	2	38	7	1	0.02	0	0	52	2.53	0.38	0.22	3.24	0	21	72	379	0.62	0.04	62
1 T peanut butter	1	3	4	8	1.6	0	0	6	0.3	0.03	0.015	2.15	0	25	107	125	0.47	0.07	12
3-inch apple	5	26	0	<1	0.56	10	9	12	0.32	0.03	0.025	0.13	0	9	202	0	0.065	0.085	5
Granola bar	1	19	2	5	0.34	0	0	29	0.72	0.08	0.05	0.14	0	21	91	78	0.42	0.03	7
2 flour tortillas	4	54	8	6	1.24	2	0	122	3.24	0.52	0.28	3.5	0	26	128	468	0.7	0.04	120
½ cup pinto beans	7	22	7	<1	0.8	0	0	41	2.22	0.16	0.08	0.34	0	47	398	2	0.92	0.13	146
1½ oz cheddar cheese	0	0	10	13	0.15	0	127	303	0.28	0.015	0.15	0.03	44	12	42	261	1.3	0.03	7.5
½ cup tomato salsa	0	8	0	<1	0.32	40	176	8	0.48	0.08	0	0.48	0	8	192	464	0.8	0.08	16
15 tortilla chips	1	17	1	8	0.36	0	6	42	0.4	0.015	0.045	0.34	0	24	53	143	0.405	0.075	3
4 small carrots (90 g)	2.5	9	1	<1	0.41	9	2531	24	0.45	0.08	0.05	0.83	0	14	291	31	0.17	0.14	12.5
2 scoops low-fat frozen yogurt	0	30	8	<1	0	2	2	274	0.14	0.06	0.32	0.16	2	26	350	106	1.34	0.08	16
1 oz almonds	3	6	6	15	6.72	0	0	74	1.02	0.06	0.22	0.94	0	83	205	3	0.82	0.03	16
TOTAL	33.5	301	74	64	13.61	135	2953	1096	16.1	2.04	1.945	16.06	258	398	3118	2696	10	1.14	577

ELLEN'S COMPLETE NUTRIENT ANALYSIS

Food	Fiber (g)	CHO (g)	Protein (g)	Fat (g)	Vitamin E (mg)	Vitamin C (mg)	Vitamin A (mcg RE)	Calcium (mg)	Iron (mg)	Thiamin (mg)	Riboflavin (mg)	Niacin (mg)	Cholesterol (mg)	Magnesium (mg)	Potassium (mg)	Sodium (mg)	Zinc (mg)	Vitamin B6 (mg)	Folate (mcg)
1 cup instant oatmeal	4	36	8	2	0.28	0	604	218	8.4	0.7	0.38	7.3	0	56	132	380	1.16	0.98	200
1 cup non-fat milk	0	12	8	<1	0.1	2	149	301	0.1	0.09	0.34	0.22	4	28	407	126	0.98	0.1	13
1½ oz raisins	3	33	0	<1	0.3	0	0	21	0.87	0.06	0.03	0.33	0	15	315	6	0.12	0.09	0
Baked potato with skin	5	51	5	<1	0.1	26	0	20	2.75	0.22	0.07	3.33	0	54	844	16	0.65	0.7	22
2 oz American cheese	0	0	12	18	0.26	0	162	344	0.22	0.02	0.2	0.04	52	12	90	800	1.68	0.04	4
3 pieces Romaine lettuce	1	1	0	<1	0.13	7	78	11	0.33	0.03	0.03	0.15	0	2	87	2	0.07	0.01	41
8 cherry tomatoes	0.5	2	0	<1	0.17	8	28	2	0.2	0.03	0.02	0.28	0	5	80	4	0.04	0.03	5
¼ cup cauliflower	0.5	1	0	<1	0.01	12	0	6	0.11	0.015	0.015	0.13	0	3	76	7	0.07	0.05	14
¼ red pepper	0	1	0	<1	0.13	35	106	2	0.08	0.01	0.005	0.01	0	2	33	0	0.02	0.04	4
1 T sunflower seeds	1	2	2	5	4.52	0	0	10	0.61	0.2	0.02	0.41	0	32	62	0	0.46	0.07	20
1 T Italian dressing	0	2	<1	7	1.56	0	4	1	0.03	0	0	0	0		2	118	0.02	0	1
8 oz orange juice	0	27	2	<1	0.47	97	20	22	0.25	0.2	0.04	0.5	0	25	473	2	0.12	0.11	109
10 small pretzels	2	47	5	2	0.13	0	0	22	2.59	0.28	0.37	3.15	0	21	88	1029	0.51	0.07	103
1 cup spaghetti noodles	4	40	7	1	0.08	0	0	10	1.96	0.29	0.14	2.34	0	25	43	1	0.74	0.05	98
1 cup canned meat sauce	8	37	8	14	5.91	26	577	68	1.94	0.13	0.17	4.51	15	60	952	1179	1.37	0.87	52
2 slices French bread	2	26	4	2	0.12	0	0	38	1.26	0.26	0.16	2.38	0	14	56	304	0.44	0.02	48
½ cup canned green beans	1	3	1	<1	0.09	3	24	18	0.61	0.01	0.04	0.14	0	9	74	178	0.2	0.02	22
1 oz pistachios	3	7	6	14	1.46	2	6	38	1.9	0.23	0.05	0.3	0	44	306	2	0.37	0.07	16
1 cup plain popcorn	1	4	1	1	0.06	0	1	1	0.14	0.02	0.01	0.12	0	9	14	29	0.23	0.01	1
TOTAL	36	332	69	66	15.88	218	1759	1153	24.35	2.795	2.09	25.64	71	416	4134	4183	9.25	3.33	773

MICHAEL'S COMPLETE NUTRIENT ANALYSIS

	Fiber (g)	CHO (g)	Protein (g)	Fat (g)	Vitamin E (mg)	Vitamin C (mg)	Vitamin A (mcg RE)	Calcium (mg)	Iron (mg)	Thiamin (mg)	Riboflavin (mg)	Niacin (mg)	Cholesterol (mg)	Magnesium (mg)	Potassium (mg)	Sodium (mg)	Zinc (mg)	Vitamin B6 (mg)	Folate (mcg)
1 toaster waffle	1	13	4	5	.53	0	25	84	.69	.08	.13	.75	39	15	91	150	.45	.04	7
8 oz fortified fat- free soy milk	1	22	6	0	ND	0	50	400	1.44	.07	.1	3	0	ND	20	60	.60	ND	24
1 cup tuna	0	19	33	19	1.95	5	55	35	2.05	.06	.14	13.7	27	39	224	514	.54	.17	16
4 slices mixed- grain bread	8	48	12	4	.64	0	0	96	3.6	.44	.36	4.56	0	56	212	508	1.32	.36	84
1 cup three bean salad	3	13	4	8	1.96	4	23	35	1.42	.07	.09	.4	0	25	224	514	.54	.04	53
Banana	3	28	1	1	.32	11	9	7	.37	.05	.12	.64	0	34	467	1	.19	.68	22
8 oz stir- fried vegetables with tofu	6.5	22	11.5	12.5	6.78	177	467	193	4.6	.32	.41	4	0	80	1033	102	1.71	.62	140
6 oz cashew chicken	1	12	37	19	1.16	2	10	36	2.9	.13	.21	14.6	88	104	460	326	2.6	.70	30
½ mango	2	17	.5	.5	1.16	28	402	10	.13	.06	.06	.6	0	10	162	2	.04	.14	15
2 cups steamed rice	2	90	8	0	.16	0	0	32	3.8	.52	.04	4.68	0	38	110	4	1.54	.30	184
8 oz hot tea	0	1	0	0	0	0	0	0	.05	0	.03	0	0	7	88	7	.05	0	12
½ cup trail mix with chocolate chips	4	32	10	24	7.8	0	4	80	2.48	.30	.16	3.22	3	118	474	88	2.3	.20	48
TOTAL	31.5	317	127	93	22.46	227	1045	1008	23.25	2.10	1.85	50.15	157	526	3565	2276	11.88	3.25	635

ND = No data available

DIETARY REFERENCE INTAKES (DRI) FOR VITAMINS

		Vitamin A (mcg RE)	Vitamin C (mg)	Vitamin D (mcg)	Vitamin E (mg)	Vitamin K (mcg)	Thiamin (mg)	Riboflavin (mg)	Niacin (mg)	Vitamin B₆ (mg)	Folate (mcg)	Vitamin B₁₂ (mcg)	Pantothenic Acid (mg)	Biotin (mcg)	Choline (mg)
Female	19-50 years	700	75	5	15	90	1.1	1.1	14	1.3	400	2.4	5	30	425
Female	51-70 years	700	75	10	15	90	1.1	1.1	14	1.5	400	2.4	5	30	425
Female	71+ years	700	75	15	15	90	1.1	1.1	14	1.5	400	2.4	5	30	425
Male	19-50 years	900	90	5	15	120	1.2	1.2	16	1.3	400	2.4	5	30	550
Male	51-70 years	900	90	10	15	120	1.2	1.2	16	1.7	400	2.4	5	30	550
Male	71+ years	900	90	15	15	120	1.2	1.2	16	1.7	400	2.4	5	30	550

Pantothenic acid, biotin, and choline are not specifically mentioned in this book. Although they are necessary vitamins, they are found widely in a variety of in foods, and deficiencies in healthy people have not been reported.

Note: This chart has been adapted and contains only adult values for males and nonpregnant females. The complete DRI are available at www.nap.edu.

Reprinted with permission from Dietary Reference Intakes for Calcium, Phosphorous, Magnesium, Vitamin D, and Fluoride (1997); Dietary Reference Intakes for Thiamin, Riboflavin, Niacin, Vitamin B₆, Folate, Vitamin B₁₂, Pantothenic Acid, Biotin, and Choline (1998); Dietary Reference Intakes for Vitamin C, Vitamin E, Selenium, and Carotenoids (2000); and Dietary Reference Intakes for Vitamin A, Vitamin K, Arsenic, Boron, Chromium, Copper, Iodine, Iron, Manganese, Molybdenum, Nickel, Silicon, Vanadium, and Zinc (2001). Copyright 2001 by the National Academy of Sciences.

DIETARY REFERENCE INTAKES (DRI) FOR MINERALS

		Calcium (mg)	Chromium (mcg)	Copper (mcg)	Fluoride (mg)	Iodine (mcg)	Iron (mg)	Magnesium (mg)	Manganese (mg)	Molybdenum (mcg)	Phosphorus (mg)	Selenium (mcg)	Zinc (mg)
Female	19-30 years	1000	25	900	3	150	18	310	1.8	45	700	55	8
Female	31-50 years	1000	25	900	3	150	18	320	1.8	45	700	55	8
Female	51-70 years	1200	20	900	3	150	8	320	1.8	45	700	55	8
Female	71+ years	1200	20	900	3	150	8	320	1.8	45	700	55	8
Male	19-30 years	1000	35	900	4	150	8	400	2.3	45	700	55	11
Male	31-50 years	1000	35	900	4	150	8	420	2.3	45	700	55	11
Male	51-70 years	1200	30	900	4	150	8	420	2.3	45	700	55	11
Male	71+ years	1200	30	900	4	150	8	420	2.3	45	700	55	11

This book has emphasized calcium and iron and includes magnesium and zinc in the nutrient analysis. The other minerals are also necessary, and they can be obtained from a variety of foods, particularly whole grains and nuts.

Note: This chart has been adapted and contains only adult values for males and nonpregnant females. The complete DRI are available at www.nap.edu.

Reprinted with permission from Dietary Reference Intakes for Calcium, Phosphorous, Magnesium, Vitamin D, and Fluoride (1997); Dietary Reference Intakes for Thiamin, Riboflavin, Niacin, Vitamin B₆, Folate, Vitamin B₁₂, Pantothenic Acid, Biotin, and Choline (1998); Dietary Reference Intakes for Vitamin C, Vitamin E, Selenium, and Carotenoids (2000); and Dietary Reference Intakes for Vitamin A, Vitamin K, Arsenic, Boron, Chromium, Copper, Iodine, Iron, Manganese, Molybdenum, Nickel, Silicon, Vanadium, and Zinc (2001). Copyright 2001 by the National Academy of Sciences.

TOLERABLE UPPER INTAKE LEVEL (UL) FOR VITAMINS

		Vitamin A (mcg RE)	Vitamin C (mg)	Vitamin D (mcg)	Vitamin E (mg)	Vitamin K (mcg)	Thiamin (mg)	Riboflavin (mg)	Niacin (mg)	Vitamin B$_6$ (mg)	Folate (mcg)	Vitamin B$_{12}$ (mcg)	Pantothenic Acid (mg)	Biotin (mcg)	Choline (mg)
Males and females	19+ years	3000	2000	50	1000	ND	ND	ND	35	100	1000	ND	ND	ND	3.5

TOLERABLE UPPER INTAKE LEVEL (UL) FOR MINERALS

		Boron (mg)	Calcium (mg)	Chromium (mcg)	Copper (mcg)	Fluoride (mg)	Iodine (mcg)	Iron (mg)	Magnesium (mg)	Manganese (mg)	Molybdenum (mcg)	Nickel (mg)	Phosphorus (mg)	Selenium (mcg)	Vanadium (mg)	Zinc (mg)
Males and females	19-70 years	20	2500	ND	10000	10	1100	45	350	11	2000	1.0	4	400	1.8	40
Males and females	71+ years	20	2500	ND	10000	10	1100	45	350	11	2000	1.0	3	400	1.8	40

Arsenic and silicon UL cannot be determined because of a lack of data but should not be added to food or supplements. Use vanadium supplements with caution. Value for magnesium is for supplements only and does not include intake from food or water.

Note: These charts have been adapted and contain only adult values for males and non-pregnant females. Some Tolerable Upper Intake Levels cannot be determined because there is a lack of data (listed in the chart as "ND"). The complete UL are available at http://www.nap.edu.

Reprinted with permission from Dietary Reference Intakes for Calcium, Phosphorous, Magnesium, Vitamin D, and Fluoride (1997); Dietary Reference Intakes for Thiamin, Riboflavin, Niacin, Vitamin B$_6$, Folate, Vitamin B$_{12}$, Pantothenic Acid, Biotin, and Choline (1998); Dietary Reference Intakes for Vitamin C, Vitamin E, Selenium, and Carotenoids (2000); and Dietary Reference Intakes for Vitamin A, Vitamin K, Arsenic, Boron, Chromium, Copper, Iodine, Iron, Manganese, Molybdenum, Nickel, Silicon, Vanadium, and Zinc (2001). Copyright 2001 by the National Academy of Sciences.

About the Author

Marie Dunford, PHD, RD, is a former professor and chair of the Department of Food Science and Nutrition at California State University, Fresno. She currently is a full-time writer and nutrition educator. Her goal is to provide unbiased nutrition information that consumers can use to make healthy food and supplement choices. She is also the author of several continuing education courses for health professionals and writes for *Today's Dietitian* magazine. Dr. Dunford lives in California with her husband and has two adult children. She is an avid tennis player and an adventuresome cook.